Sculptors and Physicians in Fifth-Century Greece

Sculptors and Physicians in Fifth-Century Greece

A Preliminary Study

GUY P.R. MÉTRAUX

McGill-Queen's University Press
Montreal & Kingston • London • Buffalo

© McGill-Queen's University Press 1995
ISBN 0-7735-1231-4
Legal deposit second quarter 1995
Bibliothèque nationale du Québec

Printed in Canada on acid-free paper

This book has been published with the help of a grant
from the Canadian Federation for the Humanities,
using funds provided by the Social Sciences and
Humanities Research Council of Canada.

McGill-Queen's University Press is grateful to the
Canada Council for support of its publishing program.

Canadian Cataloguing in Publication Data

Métraux, Guy P.R.
  Sculptors and physicians in fifth-century Greece:
  a preliminary study
  Includes bibliographical references and indexes.
  ISBN 0-7735-1231-4
  1. Sculpture, Greek. 2. Medicine and art – History. 3.
  Anatomy, Artistic – History. I. Title.
  NB94.M47 1995   733'.30938   C95-900145-X

This book was typeset by Typo Litho Composition Inc.
in 10/12 Baskerville.

Contents

Figures

Preface

This study concerns works of art, medical literature, and natural philosophy in the early classical period, from about 480 to about 450 B.C. The works of art are selected from sculpture and reliefs done in the "Severe" style, that is to say, in the principal Greek style of the generation of artists working after the Persian Wars. They include the Omphalos Apollo (plates 1–2), the funerary relief of a girl from Paros in the Metropolitan Museum of Art (plate 3), and the Riace warriors (plates 5–9). These last two statues bring the chronological series of sculptures to a close in the early high classical period, although comparative material from both earlier and later periods is used.

My selection is a sample of what seems to have been the major artistic style in this period or works of funerary art which closely reflect that style. The works differ in quality and provenance – the stele from Paros is quite different from the Omphalos Apollo (a marble copy of a bronze), and the Riace warriors are very nearly in a special category. Some of the statues are in violent motion (the Artemesion god; plate 4), others in special poses (the Delphian charioteer). The purpose of choosing these varied works is not to show their stylistic affinities. Instead, I mean to show through them some significant visual changes in the representation of the body from archaic norms; after the Persian Wars, discourse among Greek intellectuals created a culture which took on a pan-Hellenic and multivalent character, affecting works of art as much as the interpretations of life and nature. In turn, the representation of the human body in early classical works formulated the norms which we define as "classical." For that reason, understanding these works is essential to understanding what the body looked like to the Greeks, what they thought it did, and how it seemed to manifest principles of structure and function. Through these works, Greek sculptors tell us what their assumptions were about human physique and physiology and what discoveries they and others had made about them. In commissioning and installing these works, Greek patrons tell us what seemed desirable and beautiful to them and what they believed audiences would recognize and admire as plausible. By the early fifth century, what G.E.R. Lloyd has called the "inquiry into nature" had come to include evidence from the human body as well as from the visible world, and by the fourth century, conformity to "nature" became as much a standard in medicine and philosophy as it became in art.

Certain readers may well object to my discussion of so small a number of works of art, but this study is a preliminary one, not intended to cover all the phenomena of representation in the period. In addition, readers may object to my discussion of works in differing techniques and materials (marbles, bronzes, marble copies of bronzes), in differing media (sculpture in the round, reliefs, portraits), and of different provenance (Athens, Paros, and so on). I do not mean to minimize the importance of different techniques, materials, and media in Greek art, nor do I wish to mitigate the importance of local schools and styles, the discovery and recognition of which are among the most valuable products of recent scholarship. Instead, what I want to emphasize is the continuity of ideas about physique which Greek artists came to share, even though they worked in differing media and may have come from different places and been trained in slightly different traditions. In the generation (c. 480–450 B.C.) after the Persian Wars, Greek artists vastly elaborated the repertory of technical and material devices inherited from their archaic predecessors (c. 600–480 B.C.), and they worked on formulae and with styles which they changed in fundamental ways; their work led to the syntheses and varieties of art in the high classical period (c. 450–410 B.C.). I do not mean to bypass considerations such as these, that is, the varieties of media, techniques, dates, and local traditions in Greek art; but I do not think that a purely archaeological or positivistic approach is the only way to establish how works of art arose from and fitted into the contexts of their creation. All the visual arts were classed by the Greeks as *technai*, or crafts. Their practitioners – painters, sculptors, workers in terracotta, armourers, makers of decorated vases, and so on – were viewed as sharing similar mental and social environments, with little or only implicit contact with the world of ideas. But as Xenophon sought to show (see p. 3), ideas which are only implicitly present in works of art *are* ideas, and studying them can supply us with artistic intentions, motivations, and continuities which mediate between different media, techniques, and schools. What seem like marvellous and complicated varieties in the visual arts should not blind us to the interconnection among the crafts at the level of ideas, appropriated as working notions from an intellectual world itself in transition from a merely practical and descriptive to a higher, more theoretical, and more analytical one. It seems possible, then, to look at themes and issues which unite the various visual arts, rather than to emphasize their formal differences.

A study of works of art of a similar period, but in different media and techniques and from different places, is further justified by considering the relative paucity of intellectual ideas. As William Maxwell said, "The odds are on objects."[1] Relative to the abundance, variety, and geographical distribution of objects and artistic styles, ideas are few, focused, and narrowly attributable. At the same time, objects, styles, and ideas travel readily; their travelling is what we call cultural cohesion, and discovering them in expected and unexpected places allows us to recognize cultural continuities in the face of what seems, at first glance, to be a bewildering material and geographical diversity. *New* ideas are even fewer in number, and when they appear in works of art of different provenance and local style, they are worth recording. That objects and styles travel, and travelled in Greek times, needs no recapitulation: Greek philosophers and physicians were "on the road" as a matter of professional habit. Ideas, and also ideas about human physique, travelled because Greek physicians and natural philosophers travelled. The text called *Airs, Waters, Places* (or part of it, at least) is as much a physician's guidebook of the Mediterranean as it is a medical treatise; its geography is not as detailed or as accurate as Herodotus's geography in *The Persian Wars* had been, but the text is full of phrases such as "When you arrive at ..." or "When you come to ..." As such, it is prima facie evidence of the distribution, by Hippocratic physicians at least, of ideas about the body. These tended to be few in number and, as we shall see, further unified and/or subdivided by various principles, but these ideas were widely current as well, and works of art of various types can be interconnected along relatively few intellectual lines.

It is no accident that art – specifically sculpture – was classed with medicine as a *techne* by the Greeks,[2] even though physicians tried mightily to make something more of their craft. Sculpture and medicine were, in fact, the two great *technai*, and they were frequently associated with each other in ancient literature (see chapter 3). Their affinities are numerous. Both sculpture and medicine are *representational* in that they seek to represent the human body in a descriptive language, be it visual or verbal. Both are *interpretive* in that they seek to integrate visible phenomena with theoretical principles discovered rationally or intuitively. Both are *diagnostic* in that they seek to define the causes, proximate or distant, of physical manifestations and to show the visible signs (*semeia*) of these causes. The standing male nude achieved, during the early classical period, a uniformity which it had not had before; it is almost as if the sculptors anticipated what would become known as "prognosis" to the physicians, to create a somewhat uniform, predictable style, in the same way that prognosis in medicine is the prediction of inevitably recurring physical events which one physician can teach another to recognize. These affinities between sculpture and medicine required dissemination of practical and theoretical knowledge, stylistic for artists, semiological for physicians. Whether works of art are *therapeutic* is an open question, as it is an open question whether Greek medicine (apart from bandaging, bone-setting, a very few surgical procedures, and some diets) was therapeutic in the modern sense. In any case, the general parallels of sculpture and medicine are clear, and this study is devoted to establishing the specific historical contacts between the two kinded crafts.

The developments in Greek medicine from the late archaic period into the fourth century were just as interesting and just as significant as what was happening in sculpture at the same time. By the end of the fifth century, the intellectual and practical prestige of medicine, at least in the eyes of its practitioners, was assured. There were many reasons for this. The Coan school of medicine, of which the greatest exponents at the time were Hippocrates of Cos, his relatives, and his pupils, had gained a pan-Hellenic reputation. Securing that reputation involved, among many other things, the disengagement of the medical profession from popular healing traditions. This had prompted some physicians to write books and give lectures in public, activities that were prestigious and unusual at the time. Greek medical texts appeared in the fifth century and became numerous in the fourth century, apparently on the basis of an earlier body of prose works and of a well-developed verbal tradition of medical instruction, including public lectures. The forms of Greek medical texts – both literary and logical – together with their didactic intent and rhetorical strategies, sometimes kept pace with contemporary philosophical writing and incorporated its ideas or assimilated older ones. Greek medical writing and Greek philosophy develop together, and it is not possible to disengage the history of medicine from the history of natural philosophy, either intellectually or literarily. It had been a practice of natural philosophers in the sixth century to express themselves in verse or in short gnomic utterances, but by about 450 B.C., Anaxagoras of Clazomenae was writing voluminously in prose, in an apparently encylopedic form and with a coherent leading idea and a consistent intellectual procedure. He both lectured in public and had his works read aloud to audiences. In some cases, works of the Hippocratic corpus take up such forms; the physician's craft thus had as many affinities with natural philosophy as it did with its kindred craft of art.

The mediation effected, through medicine, between art and natural philosophy is the subject of this study. The connection among the three is made in the dialogue on education and virtue called the *Protagoras* (311b–c). When he came to discuss the best kind of training and education, Plato made what seemed to him a natural elision among medicine, art, and philosophy: Socrates, while in conversation with a certain young man called Hippocrates, discusses the value of an education from the young man's namesake, the famous physician of Cos. The very next people whom Socrates mentions as possible teachers for the young Hippocrates are the sculptors Polykleitos and Phidias. Art logically followed upon medicine in the philosopher's conversation, and the three – philosopher, physician, sculptor – had natural affinities in cultural expectations at the time.

The relationships among medicine, art, and natural philosophy would be easier to analyse if the dating of Greek medical treatises were as secure as that of works of art or as capable of reconstruction as the floruit of a philosopher and the first appearance of his ideas on the intellectual scene. Such is not the case. The texts of most, possibly all, medical treatises in the Hippocratic corpus have to be dated after about 400 B.C. or later. As such they are, strictly speaking, unavailable for a study of earlier art. However, the date of a text – the time at which ideas achieved literary form – most often followed the invention of the ideas contained in it by many years. It is clear that there was a considerable tradition of medical theory and culture, both anatomical and physiological, in late archaic times and throughout the fifth century. Empedocles (fl. 450 B.C.) had written on respiration, and the Pythagoreans had included considerations of the body in their speculations; indeed, the Hippocratic oath itself may well be modelled on a Pythagorean text.[3] At least one physician, Democedes of Croton, secured status as a well-paid medical official for Aegina, Athens, and Samos in the late sixth century (Herodotus *The Persian Wars* 3.125, 129–37). By the end of the fifth century, medical culture had developed in such a way as to make the intellectual and formal procedures of the later medical treatises flow directly from them. As we shall see, Anaxagoras of Clazomenae (fl. 460–430 B.C.) concerned himself with anatomical interpretation, and there was evidently a considerable tradition of medical theory which, if not written, achieved substantial verbal form as doctrine and as teaching by the second half of the fifth century. The Hippocratic oath stresses communication of knowledge from one physician to another, and the verbal *paideia* was considerable; it seems to have had a theoretical component as well as a practical one, and there is no reason to doubt that the contact between medical men and philosophers, well attested in the later medical texts themselves, did not already exist in the fifth century. Chapter 2 takes up some of the issues involved in applying medical ideas in later texts to earlier works of art.

The sharing of intellectual forms among philosophers and physicians was part of a broader alliance: medical thinkers co-opted the ideas of pre-Socratic and later natural philosophers to give structure and coherence to their works. As we shall see, medical thinking comes to be closely intertwined with natural philosophy at this time, and because the great systems of natural philosophy which came to formulation by Plato and Aristotle were in preparation earlier, understanding the pre-Socratic intellectual situation, and especially its ramifications in medical thought, tells us what the origins of the later classical systems were.

Pre-Socratic natural philosophers were concerned with the organization of matter, space, time, and animating forces and thus were concerned with the human body as well. No matter what their orientation – vitalistic, Pythagorean, monistic, Eleatic, or whatever – philosophers felt obliged to show the correspondences between cosmic structure and its manifestation in the human body. The description of the body assumed an importance in natural philosophy which it had not had in epic and lyric literature, and natural philosophers may have borrowed some of their knowledge and method from physicians.

So did the sculptors. Although Polykleitos's prose book *Kanon* (on his statue called the *Doryphoros*) has not survived, its literary form must have been based on a medical treatise or a text of natural philosophy because such were the only prose models available to him and germane to his task. In addition, sculptors of the generation previous to that of Polykleitos, those of the early classical, or Severe, style, exhibit in their statues the unmistakable influence of current medical thinking as it can be partially reconstructed from later treatises in the Hippocratic corpus and texts in natural philosophy. This influence is also the subject of the present study, and ultimately I would argue that works of art themselves constitute a record of medical thought and its diffusion – an entirely partial one, to be sure, and one which is sometimes difficult to interpret.

This study is not an illustrated medical history. Numerous such histories of great interest have been written, both by historians of science and by doctors; in these histories, works of art are mostly used as secondary sources to illustrate specific medical situations (wounds, dietary habits, instances of medical practice, and so on) without much reference to the works of art themselves. By contrast, in this study, works of art are presented as *primary* sources for information about medical attitudes, which may also be widespread attitudes based on ideas of health accepted by, or generated from, the population at large. Works of art exist, it seems to me, at an intersection where élite and popular cultures come together. Ideas about the body as represented in sculpture can combine the latest advance in natural philosophy or medicine with features which make the work of art saleable and pleasing to more traditionally minded folk (see chapters 1 and 2). For this reason, medical treatises and texts in natural philosophy are used as *secondary* evidence to investigate the sources, in both the élite and popular cultures, of ideas represented in statues. The change in the representation of human form which occurred during the early classical period and which brought to an end the stylistic norms (and also the stylistic varieties) of the archaic period and announced those of classical times was also a change in the iconography of anatomy and physiology, in the very meaning of bodily *semeia*, in Greek sculpture. The texts I have used are those that were in intellectual preparation during the fifth century and certain later texts (those of Plato and Aristotle on natural philosophy) which give direct or indirect testimony to earlier ideas. I have avoided texts of very late date or problematic intellectual origin, such as the pseudo-Hippocratic treatise *On Sevens*. In any case, the many ways in which ancient medical texts can be applied to Greek art has not been exhausted here, nor have all the works of art: the special character of the human body in Attic vase painting, for example, in relation to changes in the ideology of health will have to be broached elsewhere.

This study is an interpretive one, intended to define the area for a more complete study of ancient art and ancient medicine. The reader will become aware that there are many different ways of applying medical history to Greek and Roman art history, and for that reason I found it necessary to proceed discursively and with a more complete analysis of the medical material than is usual in a study of works of art. It goes without saying that this study is by nature interdisciplinary, and because virtually nothing has been written on the topic in this way, as far as I am aware, I have sought to suggest strategies of method for future research, both for others and for myself. The question I have sought to ask and answer is, Why does the human body look the way it does in this work of art?[4] The question is, of course, quite widely applicable.

J.J. Winckelmann, in his *History of Ancient Art* of 1764, asserted that all Graeco-Roman standing male nudes had larger left testicles than the smaller, higher ones on the right; he further made an analogy between this anatomical situation and a physiological one: the left eye had keener vision than the right one. His views on testicles in ancient sculpture cannot be confirmed, nor can his views on vision, but both notions are profoundly classicistic: Winckelmann absorbed the modes of thought of ancient writers on physique and made their view of nature his own.[5] That he was wrong, both about testicles in sculpture and testicles in human beings, is not the issue; the issue, both for him and for us, is the relation of art to nature. In most historical periods, "art" is not too hard to define. The definition of nature can be much more difficult to determine, and one of its sources is certainly current medical ideology.

In deference to the different education of modern doctors and to their post-Galenic and scientific knowledge, I have avoided referring to Greek dealers in human sickness and health as "doctors" and have instead used the term "physician," which they also would have called themselves.

To avoid undue proliferation of apparatus, I have followed the convention of placing most citations from ancient literature in the body of the text and those from modern literature in endnote form. In citing ancient texts, I have used the conventional English translations in unabbreviated form (instead of their Greek or Latin titles) for the benefit of those who might wish to consult them further. Texts of the Peripatetic school which are no longer attributed to Aristotle, but which were edited in the Teubner editions, are cited as [Aristotle] or as "pseudo-Aristotle." A listing of editions of other texts that have been used for this study is given at the beginning of the notes. An index locorum follows the bibliography.

For the spelling of Greek names, artists in general appear in English transliteration (e.g., Polykleitos), while others appear in their more widely recognized Latin transliteration (e.g., Hippocrates of Cos, Heraclitus of Ephesus).

Acknowledgments

I wish to express my gratitude to the Center for Advanced Study in the Visual Arts, National Gallery of Art, Washington, DC, for the award of an Ailsa Mellon Bruce Visiting Senior Fellowship; to the dean of the center, Professor Henry A. Millon, for his advice on an original draft and for his famous intellectual hospitality; to the staffs of the center for their assistance and patience. The staff of the library of the National Gallery of Art and the Library of Congress were most helpful, and Dorothy Hanks, of the History of Medicine Division (Surgeon-General's Collection) of the National Medical Library, National Institutes of Health, Bethesda, Md, deserves my special thanks. In 1989 Dr C. Sabbione of the Museo archeologico nazionale in Reggio di Calabria kindly allowed me to view the Riace warriors from a rolling platform. This study also benefited from a Minor Research Grant from the Fine Arts Faculty Council of York University and from the suggestions and help of a graduate student, Bonnie MacDonald.

I am grateful for the encouragement of professors William Lloyd MacDonald, Dorothy F. Glass, and Seymour Howard, as I am to the student mentioned in note 4 to the preface. This study could not have been undertaken without the help – intellectual, taxonomic, and editorial – of Dr Gudrun Kubelik-Baudler of Vienna and Prague, who has my special thanks. I have never seen a graceful way of thanking anonymous readers, whose intervention can both extend a text and prevent big and small errors from occurring. The readers for both McGill-Queen's University Press and the Canadian Federation for the Humanities were generous of their time, intelligence, and knowledge, and I thank them mightily. The blunders that remain are mine, not theirs.

My greatest thanks should have gone to my *doktor-vater*, George M.A. Hanfmann of Harvard University, who died in March 1986. Professor

Hanfmann's dissertation for admission to the philological seminar at Berlin University in 1934 was on treatises in the Hippocratic corpus. This study is dedicated to my wife, Michèle Métraux.

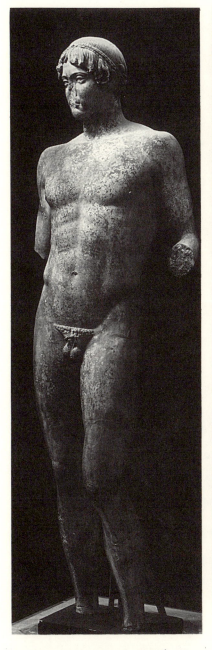 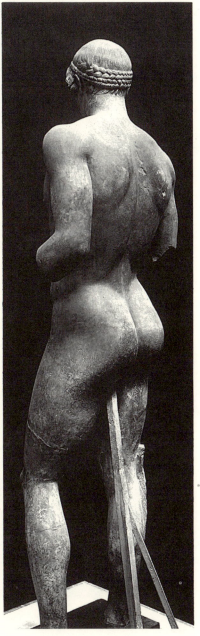

1 Omphalos Apollo, front. Roman
marble copy of a Greek original of
about 470 B.C. The veins in the upper
arms along the biceps are prominent.
Athens, National Archaeological Museum.
Photo: Alinari/Art Resource, NY.

2 Omphalos Apollo, back. Photo:
Alinari/Art Resource, NY.

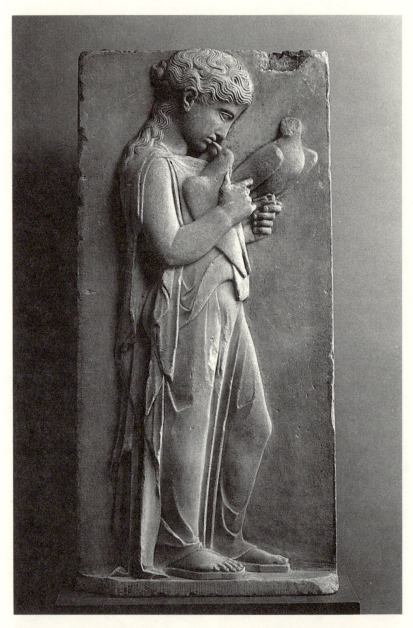

3 Funerary stele from Paros showing a young girl with her pet doves. Marble, about
470–60 B.C. The silhouette of the back and buttocks is visible because the peplos
has lost its belt; the hem of the gown has fallen over the girl's instep. New York,
Metropolitan Museum of Art. Photo: The Metropolitan Museum of Art, Fletcher
Fund, 1927 (27.45).

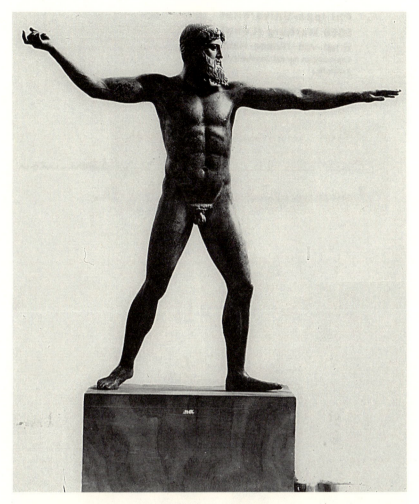

4 God from Cape Artemesion. Bronze, about 460 B.C. The veins of the arms are clearly visible. Athens, National Archaeological Museum. Photo: Foto Marburg/Art Resource, NY.

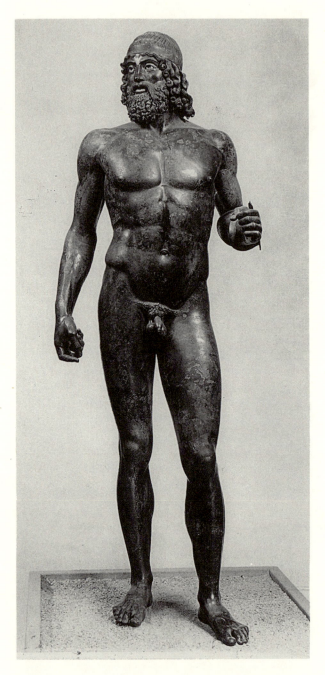

5 Riace warrior A, front. Bronze, about 460–50 B.C. Reggio
di Calabria, Museo nazionale archeologico. Photo: Alinari/
Art Resource, NY.

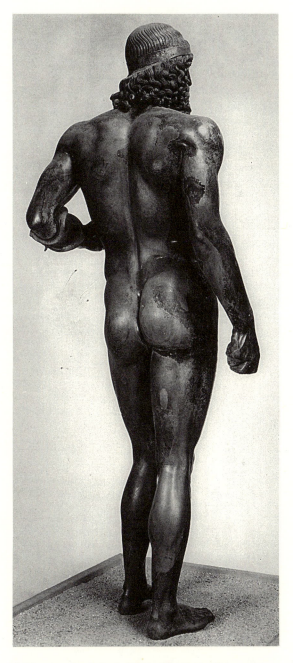

6 Riace warrior A, back. Photo: Alinari/Art Resource, NY.

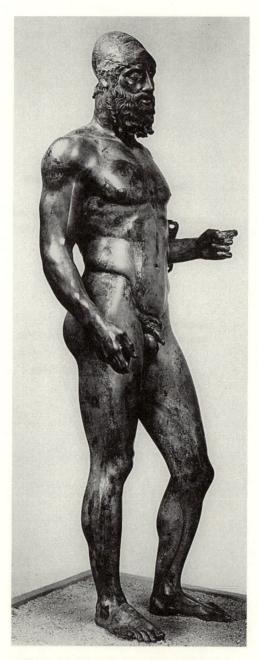

7 Riace warrior B, front. Bronze, about 460–50 B.C.
Reggio di Calabria, Museo nazionale
archeologico. Photo: Alinari/Art Resource, NY.

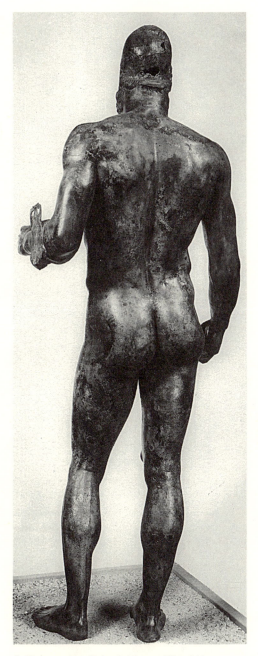

8 Riace warrior B, back. Photo: Alinari/Art
Resource, NY.

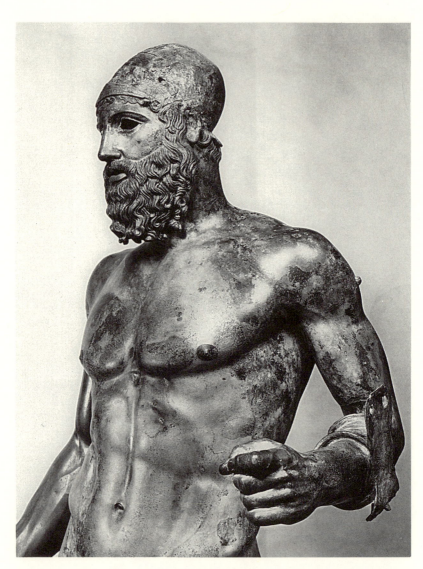

9 Riace warrior B, detail showing the veins of the abdomen. Photo: Alinari/Art Resource, NY.

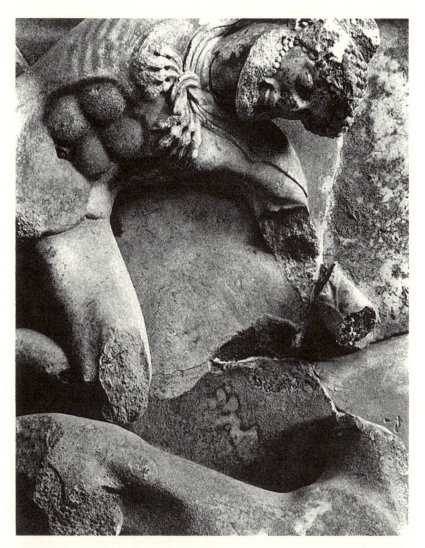

10 Metope of Heracles and the Hind of Keryneia, from the Treasury of the Athenians, Delphi, detail. Marble, about 510 B.C. Note the veins in Heracles' arm. Delphi, National Museum. Photo: Hirmer.

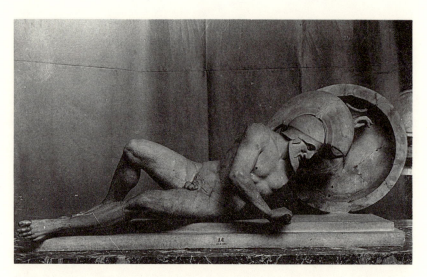

11 Dying warrior, figure O.XI from the east pediment of the Temple of Aphaea at Aegina. Marble, about 490 B.C. The veins in the left forearm have been recorded with particular emphasis by the sculptor. Munich, Glypothek. Photo: Foto Marburg/Art Resource, NY.

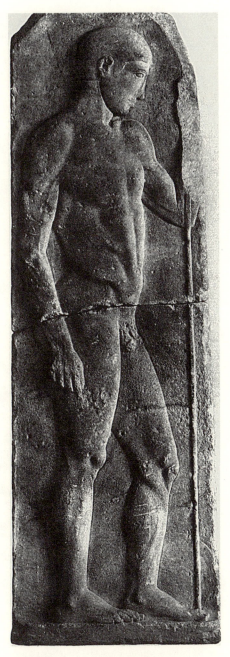

12 Funerary stele from Nisyros showing a
young man. Marble, about 470–60 B.C.
Istanbul, Archaeological Museum. Photo:
Foto Marburg/Art Resource, NY.

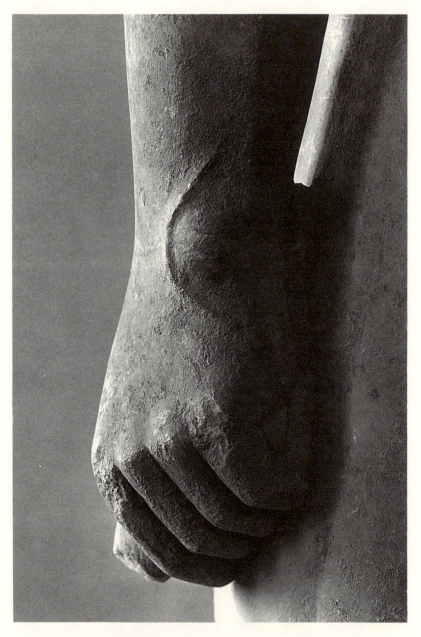

13 Metropolitan kouros, detail of hand showing phalanges and alignment of fingers. Marble. Photo: The Metropolitan Museum of Art, Fletcher Fund, 1932 (32.11.1).

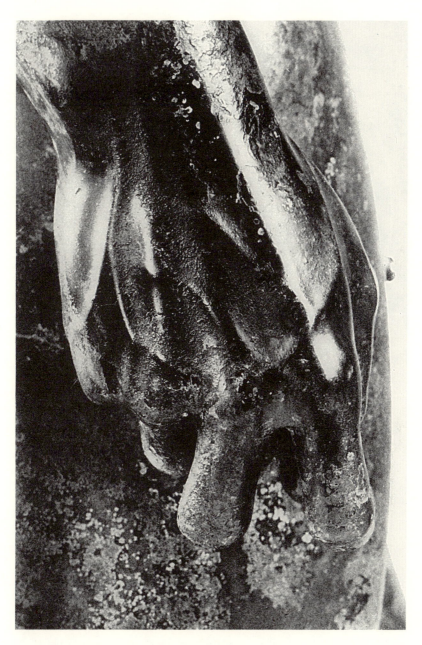

14 Riace warrior A, detail of hand. Photo: BdA.

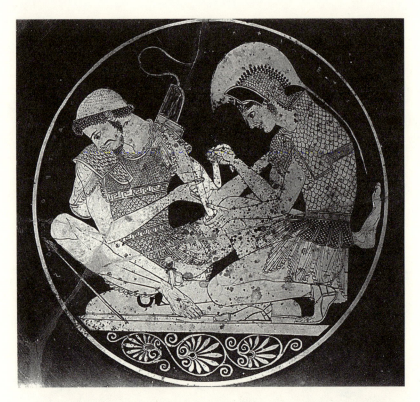

15 Sosias Painter, interior of a kylix showing Achilles bandaging Patroclus's arm. Berlin, Antikensammlungen. Photo: Foto Marburg/Art Resource, NY.

Sculptors and Physicians in Fifth-Century Greece

CHAPTER ONE

Greek Art, Medicine, and Natural Philosophy

Visiting artists' workshops put Socrates in a good mood for conversation. When he met the painter Parrhasios in his studio, they talked about how the soul's character and effects could be shown in pictures. The account continues with Socrates' skilful prompting of the sculptor Kleiton to tell us how, in his figures of athletes, he was able to represent the soul's activities by external physical features. Socrates' tone was bantering but sweet, and he was much more encouraging with the artists than he was with other people, probably because he wished to show that he too could represent the soul's activities (*ta tes psuches erga*; Xenophon *Memorabilia* 3.10.1–8).[1] Socrates' conversations with the artists have affinities with a later text called *Physiognomics*, a Peripatetic work in which the Aristotelian author tried to codify "scientifically" the relationship between external physical features and the soul.[2] Similarly, in writings by Aristotle himself, the notions of earlier philosophers and physicians (which he cites in order to refute them) and his own theories always sought to identify the soul's anatomical and physiological manifestations, in most cases very specifically; for example, dwarfs and men with large arms have bad memories, or why death can be painless ([Aristotle] *On Memory and Recollection* 453a.24–453b.4; physiology of respiration in elderly men: *On Respiration* 479a.21–4; cf. Plato *Timaeus* 81d–e). My examples are by no means extreme ones, and they are instances of an iconography of anatomy and physiology within the ideology of health (*hygieia*) in Greek culture.

With respect to the iconography of anatomy in general, its existence is not in doubt. A later instance of it can demonstrate its pervasiveness: that of "hollow" hair, with a lift or part in it at the front showing its stiffness. Plutarch tells us that both Pompey and Alexander had such hair (*anastole tes komes*; *Pompey* 2); the *anastole*, represented as a stiffness of hair around a frontal cow-lick, can be seen in a portrait of Pompey in

Copenhagen, and almost all portraits of Alexander have a rising lock of stiff hair at the peak of the forehead. The purpose of the association is clear: Plutarch wished to establish physical manifestations of the links of character between Pompey and Alexander. Scientifically speaking, in the system of physical signs (*semeia*) devised in *Physiognomics* (806b.7–11), stiff hair denoted *courage* as the soul's disposition in the person who had it (*to trikoma skleron*). There were signs of the soul's courage in the chest, shoulders, and legs as well, but the *semeion* of stiff hair persisted in the place where we would expect to find it, namely, in portrait busts. The hair lifting and/or parting slightly to display its stiffness appears in busts of Augustus and certain members of his family through Nero. I emphasize that the hair must lift or part *slightly*, because if it bristles anywhere, that is a sign of a coward (*orixon to trikoma*; 812b.28).[3]

The example raises issues of method and approach to ancient texts with respect to the history of art. The iconography of stiff hair in these portraits, like the iconography of anatomy in general, works like language and literary form – specifically like repeated variations on the same allusions or similes to link disparate persons visually and to reconcile disjointed phenomena. Plutarch did this in his coupling of Greek and Roman biographies in *Parallel Lives* (e.g., Lycurgos with Numa, Alcibiades with Coriolanus, and so on). He was writing for a cultivated audience, one which was well disposed and prepared to discover, with Plutarch's help, sets of correspondences linking famous men (of similar character, background, or political inclination) in comparable situations (moments in history, battlefields, political venues). Ultimately, the parallels between famous men showed how destiny paired and reconciled them, revealing their innate similarities without mitigating their individuality. None of Plutarch's other interpretations of physique were quite so explicit as Pompey's and Alexander's stiff hair, and he did not think that their lives were parallel, but this if anything makes his report of the physical similarity between them more telling. As an historian, he stated the facts about stiff hair in two men, and then he let his readers make up their own minds about the correspondence. Plutarch had a point to make, but he was not a propagandist.[4]

For both a cultivated audience and a less cultivated, non-literary one, portrait sculptors followed Plutarch's literary form in visual terms: they linked Alexander with Pompey, Pompey with Augustus, Augustus with Tiberius (who was not a direct blood relative), Nero with Augustus, and much later, Severus Alexander with Augustus (no relation) in stylistic ways, but also with the anatomical detail of hair lifting or parting over the forehead. Sculptors did this because it was efficient, effective, and meaningful to denote kinship of courageous soul among men who had comparable status. The hair of such men did not necessarily have to look the same to bear the *semeion* of courage. Like the repetition of similes in a panegyric speech, stiff hair helped an audience already prepared to make correspondences among portraits make them all the more quickly and precisely.[5] The capacity to understand these phenomena can be natural or cultural, or both: it is found in the natural pleasure parents take in finding family resemblances in their children (her grandmother's hands, his father's eyes, etc.) or in the social fun of a game of "Portraits" and the dangers of a game of "Animals."[6] Plutarch and the portrait sculptors developed this natural capacity in literary and visual ways because its system and meanings pre-existed in both élite and popular cultures. The soul's external manifestations was a rich field for them, and it is no surprise that authors and artists tilled it; we will find this was so in Greek sculpture as well.

Stiff hair to denote a courageous soul in portraits depends on a section of the text of *Physiognomics* which is philologically late and anyway quite inconsistent with the intellectual procedure set out at the beginning of the text because it is based almost exclusively on an analogy from animals (cowardly deer, brave lions and bears), a method of interpretation which, in the introduction to the text as we have it, is partially set aside as being too rigid and implausible an interpretive tool (805a.19–24). The inconsistency is due to a technical mistake (two separate texts were clumsily edited together), and the philological and intellectual disfigurement of this treatise is typical. Like many other ancient texts, it was modified or emended by a later Greek editor who introduced elements which tell us what and how he was thinking, independent of the original ideas of Aristotle. Such interventions in a text can be very varied and sometimes irritating, but they are not all without interest because they invest with the authority of the original thinker the ideas and observations of later or lesser writers (sometimes both).[7]

In fact, mistakes, inconsistencies, and corruptions in ancient texts can be useful for the history of culture and art because they can let us into the milieu of popular notions, common preconceptions, and the useful, life-supporting platitudes that exist in all societies. This area can be documented in works of art, in the archaeological record, and in poetry, but it is an area which Greek prose writers tended to ignore, with rare and precious exceptions. The history of Greek popular culture, both material and in terms of attitudes, is coming to be written, and it is necessary to do so because of the strength of popular culture – a kind of social and semiotic glue – in all societies.[8] For the history of art, popular culture draws together patrons, artists, and audiences of works of art into a common ambience of shared understanding and experience in which all participate to varying degrees. To be sure, this does not mean that the three types of participants did not have their own differing reactions and/or indifferences to works of art, but it is in the field where all three meet, where there is upward percolation of the popular culture into high or esoteric culture and conversely where élite ideas seep down into the popular culture, that I wish to locate my investigation of some anomalies and changes in sculpture with respect to the Greek ideology of health.[9]

In antiquity, the determination of expression in bodies, with or without clues given in the face, was a popular means of physical and psychological knowledge, no less medically or "scientifically" justifiable for also being vulgar.[10] At the élite level, Aulus Gellius tells us that Pythagoras admitted students to his discipleship only after a detailed study of their physiognomy (*Attic Nights* 1.2), and at the vulgar level, Petronius has an ordinary female attendant (*ancilla*) preferring physiognomics to other divinatory practices (*Satyricon* 126.3). Together with social behaviour categorized in typical manifestations (Theophrastus's *Characters* and the pseudo-Aristotelian *Virtues and Vices* are examples), bodily characteristics served as clues to both the state of the soul and its innate disposition, and in some further sense to its destiny. That is the point of Socrates' workshop talks with artists, and the conversations indicate that what people saw in other people, they expected to see in pictures and statues too. Today, of course, not much has changed except for the details of popular-culture physiognomics (blondes have more fun; *qui montre ses veines montre ses peines*), with one important difference: by the 350s B.C., about when the Hippocratic treatise called *Ancient Medicine* was written, attempts had already been made by professional physicians to attach cosmological and, in some cases, universal knowledge theory to the specifics of human anatomy and physiology in healthy or unhealthy states.[11] There had been a long-enduring fad for ideas. The physician who wrote *Ancient Medicine* took a very cool view of the fad; he was a person of solid common sense and disapproved of the leap from, for example, heart burn to universals, but his complaining was pointless because he was writing after at least a century during which the alliance of philosophy and medicine had been proposed and engaged and a marriage between them virtually consummated. The *mésaillance* of philosophy and medicine gives us a good idea of the irresistable intellectual glamour of philosophy throughout the later sixth and in the fifth and fourth centuries. The tone of chapter 1 of *Ancient Medicine* is sarcastic in arguing against the alliance of the two and for a return to "basics," that is, observation, discoveries made over time, tested diets (3–4), research (8), and so on. However, sarcasm is really an admission of defeat on the part of the physician. In fact, he has compromised himself in the matter anyway because the method he used in the treatise seeks to separate common, popular-culture (and also older) notions of health from his own specialized knowledge based on observation and categorization. This method – positing the popular view and attacking it in order to substitute another, more complete or more rational view – is one of the formal procedures of professional philosophical writing in antiquity and the basis of dialectic. The writer of *Ancient Medicine* borrowed the intellectual form of philosophy, thereby compromising his argument against its content and influence. His intention may have been to take advantage of the new clarity and precision of intellectual procedures and linguistic definitions which had become available in philosophy.[12] Philosophy's attraction was always its glamorous proliferation of words and definitions, and we should not be surprised at its numerous *mésaillances* with other branches of human knowledge and activity.

In addition, there is good evidence that philosophical ideas had seriously influenced popular culture – in Athens, at any rate – during the fifth century. The Sophists had become very successful and widely influential, as Socrates found out.[13] In consequence, the writer of *Ancient Medicine* was fighting philosophical ideas in medicine on two fronts: against a popular culture with a philosophical component and against an influential élite culture of philosophy. The disease of ideas was a generalized one, but apparently nowhere more virulent than in Athens, and it had resulted in Socrates' chivvying politicians, shoemakers, horse-trainers, farmers, poets, and many others for having intellectual pretensions (Plato *Apology* 22a.3ff; Xenophon *Memorabilia* 1.1.7 and 1.4.1). What Socrates found, of course, was a great variety of ideologies; he was bemused by the volatility and faddishness of notions in the popular culture, which he recognized were often glossy new surfaces on inherited ways of thinking and older ways of behaving. Ultimately, he tried to do something about them, in much the same way that the writer of *Ancient Medicine* inveighed against medical thinkers for the variety, volatility, and contradictions of their new ideas. In that sense, Socrates and the physician were doing much the same thing, that is, treating current diseases of ideas about knowledge and health.[14] They were not wrong to do so, because ideas are both volatile and conservative, and few more so than ideas about health, which were mostly prejudices, new slogans, preconceptions, old and new superstitions, bromides, and quick fixes, as the Hippocratic writers of *Ancient Medicine*, *The Art*, and *The Sacred Disease* did not hesitate to point out. The ideology of health can both change rapidly between and even within human generations and remain quite stable if it is based on the psychological habits and tastes of a society with strong traditions.

With respect to statues, what we see sometimes differs widely from what we know about their context, and this difference can raise serious issues about our understanding of them. A case in point is the impression of athletic vigour which many Greek figures project. In male nudes of the sixth and fifth centuries, there are no diseased, deformed, or emaciated figures, and hardly any obese ones either. In consequence, we assume that Greek patrons, sculptors, and audiences at all times took pleasure in looking at beautiful, healthy, athletic bodies. There is plenty of evidence that they did so, to be sure, but there is a very great danger that we will make our own cultural assumptions about the evidence, start taking certain things for granted, and thereby overlook distinctions which the Greeks themselves would have made. This is why the evidence about the ideas and notions of popular culture derived from medical writers and philosophers is important for our knowledge of Greek art: it puts us in touch with the fine and not so fine, the volatile or enduring, the wise or silly assumptions about health and other matters of physique which were current at the time. Greek health, like Greek beauty, had a history, a purpose, and a relevance to individuals and to statues which may give us clues to the interpretation of works of art.

The history of health is not always the same as the history of medicine. There are points at which they converge, but medical treatises can be quite unhelpful in documenting the history of health because Greek physicians thought it indecorous to publicize their failures and unwise to take on desperate cases (see *The Art* 8; *Prorrhetic* 2).[15] In part for that reason, all the factors – ecological, racial, dietary, sexual, social, moral, and so on – which would allow us to document Greek health fully are not always or equally discussed in medical sources, with a very few exceptions (*Airs, Waters, Places*; [Aristotle] *Problems* 949a–950a).[16] In addition, the history of health and the ideal or purpose of *good* health do not always coincide. When we are told, for example, that at Sparta there were laws requiring girls and women to exercise and compete in athletics like boys and men, and by implication to have the same food and beverage, the purpose was for the state to procure strong children and to increase the size and strength of the population for the army (Xenophon *Constitution of the Lacedaemonians* 1.3–4). Children were dieted to prevent the formation of flesh, on the theory that dieting would increase their height, and though the sentence in Xenophon's text is muddled (*Constitution* 2.9), it tells us what was thought to be flesh making: cheese, which in the Hippocratic diet is classed as "strong" (*Regimen II* 51) and which now is said to contribute to bone formation and growth in children.[17] There are many other purposes of good health; for example, in the appendix of *Rhetoric to Alexander*, the Peripatetic writer says that good health is necessary to balance the soul's vitality – health is an element in a kind of physiological politics in the body, of which the purpose was advantage for the state.[18] All of these conditions, manipulations, and idealizations of what health was or should be must have affected physique to some degree; as we shall see, in some cases these can be documented, in others not.

Turning to the health of individuals, its purpose, and its representation in statues, we come to a paradox: Greek behaviour (the time, money, resources, energy, and care spent on statues of athletes) is significantly different from certain Greek medical ideas and popular notions about the athletic condition. We have entered the milieu of interactions about art which I mentioned before, where ideas and popular notions affect and qualify patrons' motivations, artists' works, and audiences' responses. By the second half of the fifth century and intensifyingly in the fourth, philosophers on physique and professional physicians took a view of athletic conditioning which confirms, and conforms to, some very popular prejudices as well, and both of these were at some variance with Greek artistic behaviour. I begin with the philosophers and physicians and go on to sources for popular notions and then to works of art.

Both the writer who wrote the Hippocratic treatise *On Nutriment* – he was intellectually a follower of Heraclitus – and Plato agreed that the condition of the athlete is both bad and unnatural, using a word (*aphusikos*) which had a moral, as well as and a physical meaning (*On Nutriment* 34; *Republic* 410c–d).[19] In the passage cited, Plato makes clear that Socrates' interlocutors are already of the same opinion as he; they agree with him without question. The physician and the philosopher are definitive enough on the issue, but the authority of the Hippocratic *Aphorisms* (1.3) is unequivocal: athletic conditioning is dangerous and must be treated with diets and induced evacuations to reduce the flesh, and be quick about it.

These opinions on the unnatural condition of the athlete raise iconographic and perceptual problems for us. We like to think, for example, that if we could look at the original of the *Diadoumenos* of Polykleitos, that we would be sharing with the Greeks a look at a wonderfully developed athletic physique signifying, as a matter of course, things such as beauty, health, and splendid exercise. Instead, we might find that certain of our Greek companions had an unexpected distaste for such statues and regarded them as overdeveloped, unhealthy, and vulnerable. They might tell us that this body, as we see it, is in an unnatural state and must be changed; that athletic conditioning, the emblem of victory for a man, is not quite the same thing as a state of nature in the body; and that physiques in statues have little to do with being healthy.

The problem exists in poetry as well. In the late sixth century and well into the fifth, one of the major themes of poetry in the lyric tradition in which Pindar wrote was that of praising athletes and athleticism.[20] His patrons apparently paid him handsomely to write these poems. This is the agonistic celebration or theme, in which the victory of the athletes conferred honour on them and their city and memorialized their names forever. Poems and statues were accorded athletic victors: there are many examples of such commemorations. It is also in this period, and certainly by 450 B.C., that Greek iconography had developed a wide range of subjects concerned with the physique and movements of athletes.[21] Athletic themes are present in the west pediment of the temple of Zeus at Olympia, and earlier, athleticism formed a link among many Attic grave monuments from the mid-sixth century on.[22] Although the fillets which crowned many kouroi may refer to their priestly dignity, the fillet is also the sign of a victorious athlete.[23] The most famous instance of commemorative kouros figures are those of Kleobis and Biton at Delphi, dedicated to athletes who had won prizes at the Olympic games (Herodotus *Persian Wars* 1.16); there is no reason to doubt the dedication of these statues by the noblemen of Argos, even though the identity of the pair commonly cited as their originals has been questioned.[24] In addition, where notices of the lives of Greek sculptors tell us about their work – for example, in Pliny's *Natural History* – what is invariably cited is their creation of statues of athletes to honour specific victories, usually at least one such statue, if not more.[25] The date of these notices is fairly evenly distributed from the sixth through the fourth centuries and beyond. In this respect, the works of the sculptors are analogous to the poems of Pindar and must have been prompted by the same high degree of esteem for athletes as that which motivated the patrons of the poems.

It is, in fact, the athletic theme which united sculptors of the sixth century with the founders of the classical style, notably Myron and Polykleitos and in the case of the Thessalian monument and the statue of Agias at Delphi, with Lysippos and his students, who made statues for athletic and agonistic commemorations in the 330s B.C.[26] There are also considerable iconographic links from the sixth century through the fourth; one of them is the use of perfumes and pharmaceuticals by athletes, and containers for these (most often *aryballoi*) can signify both the athletic milieu and the medical one.[27] The *Apoxyomenos* athlete, based on an original by Lysippos, is removing oil and water from his body, which, in the medical terms formulated by the Aristotelian author of the *Problems*, mitigates weariness by virtue of the heat of the oil being counteracted by the moisture of the water: oil, being hot by nature, softens but then dries and hardens the skin, and so it needs water to make it penetrate better (*Problems* 881a.4–11; written about the same time as the statue was made; see also Theophrastus *On Odours* 49–50 and passim). The athlete has been using a kind of moisturizing lotion to give "deep heat relief"; the product is still on the market, available in pharmacies everywhere. The principle, of course, is that athletic effort has either cooled or heated the body excessively (there are great differences of medical opinion as to what exercise does to the body), and the hot/cold-moist/dry balance must be redressed pharmaceutically.[28]

However, the explicitness of athletic themes in sculpture presents a problem concerning how, precisely, a Greek audience would have thought about statues of bodies in a state of athletic conditioning. Of course, philosophers and physicians represent only a small part of the audience of works of art, and as far as we know, philosophers and physicians were not patrons of sculpture, but their opinions may be indicative of at least one popular view of both athletes and statues. Indeed, because Plato and the Heraclitan writer of *On Nutriment* would have disagreed on all other intellectual matters, their *rapprochement* with respect to the unnaturalness of the athlete's condition tells us that their statements were common opinions, widely held by their readers and pupils.[29] This being the case, then, at some time in the late fifth and into the fourth century, a problem arose as to how athletically conditioned bodies related to *phusis*, by which is generally meant nature and natural habit. Because the Sophists had, in the second half of the fifth century, entrenched the concept of *phusis* (nature) as opposed to *nomos* (human habit or social custom) very firmly in Athens at any rate, the conclusion presents itself that statues of athletes would have been viewed as bodies in unnatural condition because of overdevelopment. For both Plato and the Heraclitan medical writer, to be *aphusikos* represented a very serious charge, because the standard of *phusis* (or not *phusis*) was applicable a priori to all human phenomena, and it appears as such in other medical writings, notably in *Nature of Man* (2.32 and 5.22–3) and in *Regimen I* (11).[30]

So much for the philosophers of physique and the professional physicians. What of notions about athletic conditioning in popular culture? Greek behaviour (love of exercise, attendance at athletic games, commissioning of statues of athletes, and so on) should be enough to tell us what these notions were, but I would like to cite examples of written sources for the popular culture to show how they can be used.[31] Many of the sources are from the same or similar texts to those we have already looked at, but here we are looking for prejudices, bits of wisdom, preconceptions, platitudes, common sense, and truisms which percolate upward from the popular ground into élite opinion.

Plato says that athletes sleep a lot, and besides, they get sick if they depart from their diets (*Republic* 404a). Aristotle adds that they cannot stand the cold (*Problems* 887b.22–5). The vulgarity of professional coaches (*paidotribai*) was bad enough, but the writer of *Regimen I* goes on to say that they are wicked and perverse too: he implies that they are drunkards, and their profession is only a little above vendors of shoddy goods and actors (24)! These vignettes of sleepy, fussily eating athletes complaining about drafts – not to mention their despicable trainers – is given context and partially explained in *Regimen I* (35): for persons of secondary or inferior intelligence who experience difficulty in concentrating, the exercises they enjoy, such as wrestling, massage, and running (all leading to athletic conditioning), are to be strictly avoided because the enjoyment itself is unnatural and those exercises disbalance such physiques. Instead, a good bit of walking is prescribed, on the basis that it improves sight and hearing, which such persons are deficient in, and it equalizes touch, which they have "too much" of. Poor vision – vision is the noblest of the senses in all Greek medical literature – is, according to both informed opinion and popular belief, a characteristic of athletes; Aristotelian writers do not even bother to verify the truth of the proposition and just state it as a fact, even though their reason for explaining the affliction is different from that of the writer of *Regimen I* (*Problems* 958b.29–30).[32] In other words, *Regimen I*, Plato, and Aristotle all use sets of popular prejudices about athletes, namely, that their intelligence is in inverse proportion to their conditioning and that besides not being very smart, they do not see very well, sleep a lot, are dull, cannot stand the cold, and have "funny" digestion. Xenophon agreed (*Memorabilia* 3.5.13).

Whether they are argued philosophically or merely derived from notions in the popular culture, all these opinions add up, and we are left with a situation needing explanation: there is a gap between Greek thought on the athletic condition and Greek behaviour in commissioning and making (and looking at) athletically conditioned physiques in statues. Put differently, philosophers and physicians seem to be of an opposite opinion to patrons and sculptors, and the difference between them is interesting. The gap between thought on athletic conditioning and the behaviour of patrons may already have existed in the early fifth century, because intellectually the *nomos-phusis* dichotomy (the dichotomy of custom versus nature), on which all these opinions are ultimately based, appears in developed Sophistic form in the second half of the century and in an early, simpler form by the end of the sixth.[33] Later, by the fourth century, there is no question that the *nomos-phusis* dichotomy exercised an influence on taste for art, and I would go so far as to say that it was the unduly developed physique of older statues which a Peripatetic author was thinking about visually when he inveighed against older art. In a passage in *Problems* (895b.31–6) where the question concerns tameness and/or wildness in animals (*nomosphusis* again) and whether nature produces inferior animals, the writer's analogy is to the products of *technai*, first to beds and cloaks, which he says are for the most part junk nowadays – a fine early example of complaints about shoddy consumer goods – and then to old paintings and statues, which could not be in the category of excellent, but most of them in an inferior position in the not-excellent category.[34] Aristotle and his followers both recognized and participated in the volatility of visual popular culture, which quickly set aside older works of art in favour of new ones, and their fickleness is the fickleness of art consumers rather than of aesthetes or historians; this needs no recapitulation. But as the remarks imply, it is as much a change in ideas and notions about what looks "natural" (*phusikos*) in human physique that marginalizes older statues, not only their oldness. Changes in the standards and definitions of health are part of the process by which older works of art begin to look not merely old but old-fashioned.

Returning to the interesting difference of opinion and behaviour between sculptors and patrons, on the one hand, and certain philosophers and physicians, on the other, about the desirability and/or the unnatural character of athletic conditioning, what can be said specifically about the physique represented in fifth-century statues which would indicate the sculptors' views on the matter and their solutions to the problem? The nature of sculptors' commissions, that is, to make a large number of statues of athletes, had not changed significantly from the late archaic period; if anything, sculptors became more involved with athletic commissions than before. However, in what ways did the sculptors respond to this new standard in discussing physique – that it be "natural" (*phusikos*) – and at the same time satisfy their patrons and audiences with plausible representations of athletically conditioned bodies?

The answer is, I think, this: sculptors in the early fifth century began to apply a greater number of interpretive clues to the physique of their statues – veins, indices of respiration, clues to potential or actual movement, and perhaps most elusive to define, impressions of physical presence and character. The repertory of bodily gestures greatly expanded, many of them borrowed directly from athletic manoeuvres. In figures standing still, sculptors began to use *semeia*; that is, palpable or visible things like such as veins, or open mouths indicative of both speech and state of health, or characteristic stances of arms, shoulders, and legs. These were the *semeia* which physicians and philosophers were using to interpret the body: physicians to define was what normal, desirable, or in the event, symptoms of illness; philosophers with a view to defining the human body's relation to nature (*phusis*). What the sculptors did not do was to show their bodies in a special state or adaptation to a specific sport: bodies tended toward a kind of generic norm without specific marked developments of musculature or proportion, and they are characterized in general ways only. In this respect, what the sculptors did was to participate successfully in two cultures. On the one hand, they were part of the culture of athletic heroism in its élite and popular manifestations, and this was a source of patronage and opportunities for them. On the other hand, they participated in a medical and philosophical culture which had begun, already in the fifth century, to develop some distaste for the professionalism of sport and the physique and pretensions of athletes on the basis of new standards of nature. The sculptors made it their business to stay abreast of the new standards, and they applied current ideas about physique to their statues' bodies, making broad fields for interpretive codes and ideas, without at the same time trying to portray any given physique or to typify physique with respect to the effects of a specific training or exercise on it. They seem to have wished, like the physicians, to reduce the body to a normal state of nature, to be *phusikos*.[35]

How the bodily clues, or *semeia*, were interpreted is, of course, not the same in every case. While philosophers and physicians unite in certain opinions and in using certain popular prejudices about the body, they divide on other matters, the most important being the interpretation of individual physiques. All other things being equal, writers in the Hippocratic corpus stress the great variety and individuality of human anatomy, physiology, and disease, as well they should if they were practising physicians, and even if they were not, they were sufficiently alert to clinical considerations to do so. Greek physicians generalized about the body, categorizing their observations toward a norm, and for the most part, though not always, they avoided the type of technical philosophic argumentation called *hupothesis*, that is, arguing from unverified propositions arrived at by dialectical argument.[36] The tradition of medical thinking and rhetoric, as it is represented in later treatises, always mustered clinical observation and the interpretation of bodily *semeia* as the basis for making statements about "normal" nature and a "normal" body. An example is the argumentation in the *Sacred Disease*, in which the illness is viewed entirely as a sporadic, but explainable, deviation from the normal state.

In contrast to the physicians, the philosophers – Empedocles, Plato, and Aristotle – did not just generalize: they saw divine origins and universal laws of motion and causation in their observations, facts, and notions about the body. This eagerness to "see through" the body to universal principles is part of philosophers' tendency to create a teleology of the body, in which all aspects of anatomy and physiology are relatable to other, higher and primordial causes. The most elevated expression of this teleology, admittedly presented as probable rather than actual, is the anatomy and physiology of man in the *Timaeus*; the most temperate expression of the teleological tendency is in Aristotle, particularly in his *Movement of Animals* and *Progression of Animals*, but the differences between Plato's teleology of the body and Aristotle's are only matters of degree and taste, not any fundamental difference of approach.[37] This raises the question of how male nudes – where narrative or iconographic elements were not specially prominent – were represented before the late fourth century B.C.: were bodies represented as generalized according to the ways in which the body was described in medical literature, or were they meant to be "seen through" in some teleological way, to reflect divine origins and causation, in the manner of the philosophers? The question is applicable to statues made before about 350 B.C., I think, because by the mid-fourth century there are, *mutatis mutandis*, indications that beauty, as a divine idea, could compositely or uniquely be put into a statue, either by building up beautiful individual parts or by the achievements of inspired artistic talent or in line with professional art criticism, and "seeing through" teleologically became, for some spectators, an accepted way of looking at works of art.[38] But prior to these developments, in the archaic and earlier classical periods, the alternatives of generalization toward a norm or a teleological "seeing through" present themselves on the model of the differences between medicine and philosophy. And because generalization and teleological interpretation are quite different propositions about human physique, in statues as much as in medical and philosophical thought, we must take the writers seriously and ultimately answer the question, even though it can be only partially answered here (see chapter 4).

Thus Greek statues of athletes, when set in relation to notions about the physical and moral development of athletes among physicians and philosophers, exhibit something of these attitudes, even though they are also part of the big cultural investment in praising athleticism. This duality seems anomalous, but only if we say that Greek sculptors were merely reflecting ideas from other, higher, more intellectual and/or richer (patronal) milieux in their own society. Such cannot have been the case: sculptors created a satisfactory visual culture of their own, intentionally appropriating what they needed from what was current. In any case, all complex societies exhibit such anomalies or inconsistencies; no special explanation of them is needed. More serious are the problems which arise while investigating them. The main one, to my mind, is this: how were ideas applied to works of art, specifically ideas in medicine and in the various interpretations of the body, and in what way or to what extent did sculptors adopt and adapt these ideas and interpretations for their own purposes? The problem is only partially a technical issue of Greek source texts in medicine and natural philosophy; there are historical and methodological ones as well, and they involve the documentation of ideas in the fifth century. The following chapter incorporates some of the answers to the question.

CHAPTER TWO

Statues and Texts

The objection may be legitimately raised that, because ideas in the high culture and notions in the popular culture are volatile, it is improper to apply any anatomical or physiological concept to any work of art before the concept appears in writings to which dates can be assigned, in most cases not much before about 400 B.C. In other words, concepts whose first appearance in written form is later cannot be used to interpret earlier works of art. The objection is by no means merely hypothetical and must be answered.

In order to do so, I present three areas of relationship to establish some of the standards by which medical ideas about the body and certain philosophical notions can be satisfactorily applied to early classical works of art. In addition, there are issues and topics in medical treatises of which the relevance to works of art in the fifth century needs some discussion, and there are some fourth-century medical and philosophical concerns which have to be set aside as irrelevant to early classical art, most notably the concept of the soul and its promptings to the body. Ideas about the soul were in maturation only in the second half of the fifth century, and what the alternatives of interpretation or intent might have been needs to be broached here and in subsequent chapters. Pre-Socratic philosophers had ideas of animating forces in the body, but the concept of the soul as devised by Socrates and codified by Plato was as yet in the future.

A: MEDICAL TEXTS AND GREEK ARTISTIC CULTURE

Greek medical writing, as a separate category of literary enterprise, was practised with any regularity only in the fourth century, though some treatises of the Hippocratic corpus may date from the very late fifth century. This does not mean, however, that there had not been occasions for systematic medical investigation, prompted in part by the eagerness among pre-Socratic philosopers to explain the causes of natural phenomena and especially to explain or set aside popular beliefs. Conventional ideas about the body and health are an especially deep-seated part of human culture, in part because there are few ways of proving what the body does. Even in societies well equipped with media, educational institutions, and a tradition of scientific investigation, and to a much greater extent in cultures with no science in the modern definition, human beings do not know very much about their own anatomy. We know even less about our physiology. We must guess at the structure of the internal parts of our bodies, at the causes and purposes of organs and functions, or else we must be told about them; there is little that is "natural" or merely obvious about our knowledge of our bodies. Guessing is good, but there are many better ways of learning: the traditions of a family, a grandfather, or a kinship group or local community; the opinion of a priest or consultation with a religious healing centre; the standards of health and diet legislated by the state, as at Sparta, or reinforced by age group; class affiliation; the lore and norms of sex and age groups; working conditions and environment; one's own trial-and-error experiments with diet and exercise; and the advice of experts, who may be quacks, late learners, snake-oil hucksters, faddists (cf. Plato *Republic* 406d–407e), or mediocre doctors, or physicians of intelligence, experience, and justified reputation. Ultimately, one may wish also to consult a soul doctor (*psuche-iatros*) such as Socrates. The sources of knowledge about the body are embedded in traditional social structures and environments, and this kind of knowledge about health necessarily shares both the resistance to change of such structures – their enduring character – and also their changeability and adaptability – their elastic social suppleness to endure over time.[1]

To be sure, this kind of knowledge was very rarely recorded because it was verbally transmitted. But that does not mean there were not old questions about health to which various answers were given, or new questions to which answers were also given, in the popular culture.[2] A parallel modern question is, Why do we say "God bless you" when someone sneezes? When questions such as these surfaced in recorded form in medical texts and elsewhere, it took the combined experience and intellectual ingenuity of almost every Hippocratic writer and many philosophers (including Plato and Aristotle) to elucidate the matter. Explaining sneezing was indispensable to almost all Greek medical investigation and almost all philosophical writing about physique; sneezing is very interesting, since it is universal in humans, common and mysterious at the same time.[3] The explanations vary, of course, but the fact that they keep recurring indicates that the question itself was of long standing in the popular mind, one to which professionals were bound to supply an answer. Otherwise, their ideas could not be plausible, and it is only if sneezing were plausibly explained that the explanation of many other things would work; for example, explanations for why we are right-handed, what goes on in the stomach, why men shudder when they urinate, why we do not have lower ribs, where the soul is or is not, what respiration might be for, and so on. It is obvious from the difference in degree of importance of what is explained to us by Greek physicians and natural philosophers when they come to analyse the body that prevailing ignorance and popular beliefs about physique and physiology were real, various, numerous, and long established. The difference between sneezing and shuddering is almost as precisely and completely treated in medical and philosophical treatises as the location of the soul, and I would suggest that such precision and completeness, documentable in written form as of the mid-fourth century (from *Ancient Medicine* to Aristotle) cannot merely have begun at that time; why we sneeze and shudder, and many other anatomical and physiological questions, must have been asked earlier, and answers been given. Aristotle and his followers, for example, are anxious to point out that sneezing is *not* of divine origin, and the context of their explanation indicates that they are refuting some enduring popular misconceptions which claimed that it *was* (*History of Animals* 492b.8; [Aristotle] *Problems* 962a.21–4). In sum, it is the kinds of questions answered in the texts – the simplicity and commonplace character of the questions and the completeness and pertinacity of the answers – that allow us to use later concepts, questions, and explanations (partial or complete) to elucidate earlier works of art; questions endure, given the nature of the society and the popular culture from which they come. After all, the patrons, artists, and audience of statues were the same people who were asking about sneezing and many other things. For this reason, medical texts and later explanations by natural philosophers are germane to earlier works of art and may properly be juxtaposed with them, because they answer questions which were not, in many cases, new ones. Fourth-century medical texts thus represent a repository for earlier medical thinking.

The situation is further illustrated by the appearance, on statues representing nude males, of blood vessels. The appearance of superficial veins occurs in the early fifth century. The veins are not necessarily represented on all statues in the period after about 490 through the 430s B.C., and while the ones shown are fairly consistent, there are variations among them which might have had a special significance for their sculptors. But they do appear, and while the reasons for their appearance is the subject of chapter 3, the question can be asked: What, in the medical culture of the fifth and fourth centuries, might the precocious appearance of blood vessels on statues mean when physicians' concern about blood in the body achieves literary form (in medical texts) only well after the statues, sometimes as much as a century after? For example, the treatise *Nature of Man*, in which the origins, functions, sizes, and map of the "pairs" of blood vessels are very specifically described, gives a picture of blood in the body which, as we shall see, is represented with an astonishing accuracy by the sculptors of the Riace bronze warriors around 450 B.C., perhaps sixty years or even more before the treatise came to be put together.[4] It is certainly not the case that artists would have arbitrarily added an anatomical feature to their works without reason, nor would an improved naturalism in sculpture necessarily dictate the addition of particular superficial veins: at the time, there were other devices of naturalism, in some cases more obvious ones, and of course there were other superficial veins which could have been chosen for sculptural emphasis.[5]

The apparently anachronistic relationship of art and medicine regarding superficial veins and other matters can be partially resolved by considering the character and nature of Greek medicine as a rational inquiry. As G.E.R. Lloyd has recently pointed out, the elements of originality and what he calls "egotism" in scientific treatises betray the existence of lively traditions of medical thinking and observation that were old by at least a century and a half. Indeed, a continual rivalry among thinkers – and we have no reason to exclude physicians from this category – seems to have been the norm since at least the end of the sixth century. So much was this so that when medical thinking was committed to writing, a combative tone was often adopted as a matter of course, and commentators could be expected to write voluminously on any given treatise, in its defence or to attack it. The combative and competitive tone of medical writing comes from one of its original forms in the fifth century, namely, public lectures or declamations given by physicians at Olympia with the intention of disseminating new ideas persuasively to a mixed audience. If this is the case, sculptors at work on commissions at Olympia would have been in the audience.[6] In addition, medicine had a considerable *paideia* and a tradition of close training of one physician by another, and in that respect, it may have had a system of intellectual affiliations not dissimilar to the Pythagorean brotherhood or the Sophistic education. For these reasons, a consistent and enduring tradition of ideas and observations – and a body of empirical data structured in ways which were germane to current or concurrent intellectual principles – had been developed by physicians in the fifth century. While the development of an opposition between the medical "schools" of Cnidos and Cos may have been exaggerated for rhetorical and literary reasons in the fourth century, there seems no particular reason to doubt the existence of groups of physicians who found themselves in substantial intellectual disagreement with each other and in vivid competition to promote their own views successfully and extend their influence.[7] The situation of disagreement and competition among thinkers of scientific disposition – physicians as well as philosophers – can perhaps be seen as arising from the continual contact which they had with folk beliefs, lore, and practices.[8]

What was committed to writing in medical treatises in the fourth century was in part the residue of medical opinion, teaching, and observation already developed in the fifth, and there is no reason to think that what was written about during the fourth century had not been under discussion – granted, in probably quite different ways and with different intellectual intentions – throughout the preceding century.[9] For artists in the fifth century, the representation of blood vessels can certainly signify a *paideia* from physicians. As we shall see, there were available to them at least three quite different interpretations of the vascular system – at least as many as those which appear in fourth-century treatises – and perhaps even more, because not all that was thought about earlier was written down later. For example, Loxus, a physician-physiognomist of the late fifth century, had taught that blood was the seat of the soul and that the blood vessels were signs of its character and health. This was a *paideia* which Loxus had developed from the earlier teachings of Empedocles and Critias (*Anon.Lat. Physiognomonia* 1.2; cf. Cicero *Tusculan Disputations* 1.19 and Tertullian *On the Soul* 5.2).[10] Loxus' ideas on blood and blood vessels were not reproduced in the same way in subsequent medical treatises: by the time medical treatises came to be written in the fourth century, the basis of opinion about the location of the soul in the body had changed, and the soul's character (under the influence of Socrates' and Plato's teaching on the matter) had developed in a such a way as to separate soul from blood or any other material thing, which would by then have been viewed as either too specific a medium or irrelevant. Still, Loxus' idea about blood had been "in circulation" in the fifth century. The fact that it did not survive to be written down in a medical treatise does not mean that similar ideas by his contemporaries and predecessors did not find their way into other medical texts. Since blood and its interpretation were matters of principled disputation, the appearance of blood vessels in statues of the fifth century indicates, at the very least, that medical and philosophical ideas were circulating in élite intellectual circles and in artists' workshops.

It is for this reason that, in a limited way, works of art can be used for purposes of revealing current thinking about physique at times when written sources on the topic are absent or silent. I stress in a *limited* way because works of art are not a good substitute for the discourse of medical treatises, and statues do not have the detailed interpretative code of description and analysis which is possible only in a literary argument and in a verbal exchange. On the other hand, works of art, especially when they exhibit a change toward a new systematic representation of bodily characteristics that had been absent in earlier works, can alert us to the framework (if not the details) of informed discussion about the body. It is precisely this informed discussion which physicians engaged in and which, I believe, sculptors came to pay some attention to. Moreover, sculptors need neither have believed nor have understood the precise intellectual intentions of the physicians, which in any case would have been fairly irrelevant to their own tasks and interests. The teachings of physicians were available to sculptors – as fashion, as fad, or as stimulus for research in artistic representation. The evidence to be presented here will show that medical ideas were known to artists, not as specific sources but as a context for representation. No exaggerated claim to an intimate and lively participation in the world of ideas need be advanced for artists, but as we shall see, at least one element of anatomy – the hand – developed a design by sculptors in the fifth century which may have been derived from Anaxagoras's lecturing at Athens in the years between about 460 and 430 B.C. While he did ultimately write an encyclopedia, we cannot know and have every reason to doubt that any artist would have read it. On the contrary, Anaxagoras was famous primarily for his public teaching at Athens, and the model of his instruction may well have been that followed by physicians. His ideas in lecture form would have been available to artists as well, and Pericles, the friend and patron of sculptors, was also Anaxagoras's friend, pupil, patron, and protector.

A culture is no less a culture for not being literary, and an intellectual context is no less of one for not manifesting the varieties of its teaching – its agreements and its disagreements – in written forms. Not all medical situations of the fifth century were reproduced in fourth-century treatises, but because medicine had become highly philosophical early on, there is a good check against later intrusions into medical thought: it is possible to set aside or qualify, as need be, concepts which are of a later date or of a different origin. One of these concepts, which is often included in medical treatises, is that of "soul" in its Platonic or

Aristotelian – ultimately, in its Socratic – formulae. There were alternatives to the Socratic definitions of soul in pre-Socratic philosophy and medical theory, and when we turn to the medical texts themselves, we must, of course, also set aside concepts associated with discoveries which were definitely fourth-century or Hellenistic ones, such as that of the nerves. An intellectual context can be reconstructed on the basis of its later manifestations in literary form, but elements such as soul and nerves which were developed later have to be set aside.

With regard to artistic culture, of course, the situation is quite different from an intellectual culture which did not manifest itself in literary form. There is no art without works of it, and in this respect sculpture can embody ideas, in most cases indirectly and for its own purposes, in ways which are a notation of the concerns and preoccupations of intellectuals. Natural philosophy may have little capacity for being reproduced in works of art. By contrast, knowledge and interpretation of anatomy and physiology certainly can be represented both visually in works of art and verbally in interpretive accounts. To the extent that the emphases and the colouring of "facts" about the body are themselves subject to philosophical manipulation and mutation, works of art may very well tell us, in indirect ways, what people have been thinking. For this reason, medical texts can indeed bear, with reservations for anachronisms, on works of art.[11]

B: STATUES AND NATURE

Medicine and sculpture are both, in quite different ways, investigations of nature; lively or unexpected change in either one means that the definitions of nature – we might say, the nature of nature – are undergoing change. There was certainly nothing monolithic about classical culture, either intellectually or artistically, but the diversity of its products should not blind us to a certain unanimity of approach which gives cohesion to the work of Greek sculptors in the fifth century. Equally, the investigation of nature and body by natural philosophers and physicians did not create much in the way of consensus as such, but a certain unanimity came about, if only on very generalized terms – agreeing to discuss blood and respiration, for example, or the source and nature of human motion. For this reason, the parallel unanimities of medicine, natural philosophy, and works of art in the fifth century can be investigated, and indeed, statues can sometimes provide clues to what people might be thinking about in other areas of intellectual concern. Statues, the means of their patronage, and the technical conditions under which they were made exhibit enduring characteristics – and some slow changes – similar to the endurance of questions (and answers) about physique and physiology, such as sneezing. There are many features of physique in statues which change from the early sixth through the mid-fifth century, and the changes in style were very great, of course, but assumptions about the body endure and provide genuine links between early kouroi and many later works. The linkage is not necessarily stylistic but more in terms of the values which physique in Greek statues exhibits. The exception is the head, which changes rapidly at certain times and very slowly at others. But in general, it is impossible that statues could have been made by artists, accepted by patrons, and thought plausible (not to mention beautiful) by an audience if they did not correspond at some level to contemporary anatomical and physiological thinking in the popular and/or élite culture. This is what is called public taste, part of a general *vox populi* in artistic matters. I cite the *size* of Greek statues as an example of agreement, consistency, and continuity, in part formed by medical and philosophical ideas.

Some (not all) kouros figures in the early sixth century are of colossal size or very much larger than life-size. But these large statues ceased to be made, except very sporadically, about 560–550 B.C. (some are unfinished). After that, male nudes came to be represented in statues life-sized or only a little larger.[12] Of course, in this period there were many variables. For example, the large number of Attic kouroi dedicated soon after the entrenchment of Pisistratus's tyranny about 540 B.C. plainly indicates that patrons, or a greater number of patrons, felt it necessary to commission them, thereby increasing demand, to which sculptors could respond by reducing the size of statues to streamline production and cut costs as necessary (if there were a greater number of relatively less wealthy patrons and/or less time to produce a larger number of statues).[13] In addition, the widespread construction of stone temples in the second half of the sixth century may have constituted a competition for expenditure (in the form of voluntary or involuntary subscriptions to building funds by patrons who otherwise might have commissioned kouroi) or for manpower (sculptors finding better, steadier, more interesting, more prestigious and/or more lucrative work on building sites), thereby necessitating a streamlining of production by reducing the size of statues (this would not, however, explain the greater abundance of kouroi).[14] Either or both of these explanations, which are economic and practical ones, do not set aside others; the necessity for making smaller statues could also have been a matter of popular taste, corresponding to an existing demand for plausibly sized statues. In any of these cases, Greek behaviour in the matter of size of statues is pretty consistent through the sixth century and into the fifth: statues become smaller, gravitating toward life-size.

Certainly by the mid-fifth century, any statue much bigger than life-size was either iconographically or technically special or both, as in the case of the three colossi in ivory and gold, one by Polykleitos (Hera of Argos), the other two by Phidias (Athena Parthenos, Zeus of Olympia), or else it was in an architectural setting viewed under specific conditions (Athena Promachos of Phidias on the Athenian Acropolis or pedimental sculpture).[15] The point is that the standard of anatomical plausibility is satisfied by appropriateness of size in statues, whatever other reasons there may have been. I am assuming that to Greek patrons and audiences, life-sized or slightly over life-sized statues were more plausible, as figures and as works of art, than much bigger ones. Such, in any case, is the intellectual principle of the Hippocratic aphorism "A large body is noble and not unpleasing in a youth; it is not appropriate and less desirable than a smaller body in old age" (*Aphorisms* 1.54).[16] The morality of this aphorism is like Solon's dictum "Keep the end of everything in mind" (Herodotus *Persian Wars* 1.32); it is also an example of a physician generalizing toward a commonly held physical and moral norm, in this case a taste for "normal" sizes in bodies and "normal" sizes in moral attitudes. There is no reason to think that Hippocrates was uninfluenced by common opinions in the popular and patronal culture, in which a preference for life-sized bodies had expressed itself in statue commissions well before his day. In another context, issues of size in human bodies are addressed much later (third century B.C.) in *Physiognomics* (813b.7–9), where small size in men denoted alertness and quick reactions because the blood, which transmits perceptions from the organs of sense, did not have so far to go to return to the seat of the soul in the upper torso. Large-bodied men's blood had a greater way to go, so they are duller. Thus, plausibility with respect to statues which are life-sized or or only a little bigger guarantees that we are looking at alert, reactive figures. For this reason, the medical teaching, itself surfacing in written form in medical texts, provided a context for statues – in this case, the size of statues – about a century or more before the professional physicians happened to write down the reasons why "normally" sized bodies are good ones. Thus, it seems not impossible to discuss medical ideas in works of art, even though their written form might be later than a given statue.

The issue of size in human bodies and in statues raises a question of naturalism in sculpture which is similar to that of the superficial veins. The question is one which I would call that of "matching up," and it involves methodological issues about Greek art – all figural art, in fact – which cannot be fully examined here. The question, simply put, is this: Can we say that the improved naturalism of Greek sculpture in the fifth century B.C. was a result of sculptors mechanically "matching up" human bodies with their models?[17] This would put sculptors at the level of limners, "going over the lines" of human faces and bodily features, with something of the same results as limners' portraits: a repetitious sameness within an apparent, but meaningless, variety of individual traits.[18] The chaotic result would have been a series of body portraits, and it is clear from the uniformities and similarities among male standing nudes of the classical period that such "matching up" was not the case at all.[19] Rather, by the fifth century, and certainly by the fourth, the movement toward an improved naturalism was the result of sculptors assimilating theoretical, or what we could call aesthetic, ideas, such as the desire to show the operation of mind or the activities of the soul, which Socrates talked about with Parrhasios the painter and Kleiton the sculptor (see above, p. off.), or a perfected beauty, as in the *Doryphoros* of Polykleitos, and so on. Sculptors were prompted toward naturalism by ideas, and while the sources of their ideas are not always accurately identifiable in the fifth century, the potent effect of ideas on works of art is registerable at least.[20] It can further be noted that philosophers proceeded in similar fashion, with the enunciation of a principle or set of principles, which in turn explained and predicted the behaviour of matter, of motion, of structure both bodily and cosmic, and so on; the point is that "matching up," if it occured at all, was an entirely secondary process, independent of the promptings toward improvements in naturalism such as blood vessels.[21] In chapter 3, I will show that sculptors, far from "matching up," gave themselves over to a selective, highly specialized, and only partially accurate representation of blood vessels. Their accuracy, such as it was, was based on quite different considerations – considerations of medical theory.

What the ideas were which prompted sculptors to begin depicting blood vessels in human figures will be discussed presently. However, a point should be made here which settles the issue of "matching up" as the basis of naturalism in Greek sculpture. Blood vessels, which had not appeared in plastic form in sixth-century and early-fifth-century depictions of human beings, *did* appear in certain depictions of animals, even though these are rare and the examples, as far as I am aware, are horses (or the equine parts of centaurs) exclusively. Blood vessels are shown on the muzzle of a prancing horse in a relief from the Athenian Acropolis of the late sixth century and on the bellies of horses and centaurs on the pediments at Olympia. Later, they appear with great prominence on the centaurs of the Parthenon metopes and on the horses of the Parthenon frieze, though by no means on all.[22] Thus, sculptors were aware of blood vessels, they knew how to depict them, and in some few instances, were willing to do so, as far as their interests and talents allowed. In situations where active poses or poses anticipating action were to be shown (as in the pediments of the Zeus temple at Olympia), they did not hesitate to apply their knowledge of nature from what they could observe. However, for sculptors, depicting blood vessels in the *human* body seems to have required a different kind of prompting, one which was of greater force and needed to be more systematic than what could be learned from visual observation. By the mid-fifth century, as we shall see, there are documentable instances of natural philosophers and physicians providing systems whereby blood vessels could be understood, justified, mapped, differentiated, and related to other parts of bodily systems; these systems go well beyond visual observation and enter the realm of interpretive anatomy and speculation about physiology. Philosophers and physicians had developed theories of blood vessels by the late sixth century. These theories, I think, were the promptings for sculptors to select which blood vessels to show, when to show them, and conversely, where not to do so, on human figures. Sculptors were responding to the discoveries and theories about nature which medical practitioners and other intellectuals were already investigating.[23] That written texts postdate the statues which exhibit some of the results of these contemporary investigations does not matter: the statues themselves are a partial record of the activity.

C: STATUES AND MEDICAL WRITING

Certain linguistic and intellectual characteristics make later medical treatises and texts in natural philosophy available to interpret earlier works of art. By any reckoning, Greek medical treatises are extremely interdependent, despite large differences among them.[24] Even if we grant inadequacies of method, taxonomy, and accurate nomenclature (Aristotle often says, in *Parts of Animals* and *History of Animals*, that there is "no special word" for whatever he is describing), and if we set aside inadequacies of diagnostic procedure (already criticized in antiquity) if we take into account the absence of all modern questions and equipment, Hippocratic medicine and Greek philosophy of human physique remain ideological, even in the most optimistic assessment.[25] The content of the Hippocratic treatises is very varied, and some of them contain large amounts of carefully presented clinical reports, some are lists and aphoristic collections of various kinds, many are essays in developed literary forms, others are diet books, prescription formulae, studies of specific issues in gynecology, dislocations, and so on. In style, they also vary; in readership, they are differently aimed; in knowledge theory and philosophy of nature, they almost never agree. However, to make a large generalization, the Hippocratic treatises and the natural philosophers' writings contained, in part, two kinds of information: interpretations from observations (or things presented as observations) and repetitions (or variations on the latter in the form of special pleadings, prejudices, platitudes, and so on).[26] Interpretations from observations can occasionally be fairly accurately dated, as, for example, the diagrams to seven lost books called *Dissections*, written by Aristotle in the 340s or 330s to which he refers frequently in his *History of Animals*.[27] But in many instances, interpretations from observations cannot be accurately dated at all because the observations themselves are merely restatements or adaptations from previous medical writings. Such is the case in *On Nutriment* of about 300 B.C., in which the principle of interpretation and the interpretations themselves are based on observations made by Heraclitus of Ephesus, who lived about one hundred and fifty years before the treatise was written.[28] Thus, unless observations can be incontrovertably proved to have been made by the writer of a given treatise, we cannot assume that the observations set before us are his; they may be the earlier opinions of others, or adaptations of earlier interpretations, or interpretations disguised as observations, or pieces of special pleading, and so on.

Another, by no means infrequent, kind of information in medical writings is repetition, sometimes of nothing more than inherited platitudes.[29] Nonsense is endemic, and it can be old or new or of any date, but the context in which it appears can sometimes verify its persistence and thus its longevity. When Aristotle tells us, for example, that "men with flat feet are mischievous," there is *no* reason to think that he is joking; rather, the relative paucity of such remarks indicates, if anything, that they were common interpretations which, or the like of which, were current, plausible, and had been believed for a long time (*History of Animals* 494a.16–17). Aristotle included them because he had to; their currency and enduring popularity made their inclusion indispensable. This is not to say that kouroi with flat feet represent men who were mischievous practical jokers (or, conversely, that ones with well-arched feet are of a serious disposition); rather, it is the tendency toward such kinds of interpretations to which we must be alert, and we can use them where statues exhibit extreme and abundant correspondences among themselves or when significant changes in details (such as flat-footedness) occur. Used with caution, such evidence can serve as an interpretive tool because it can usefully reveal what people believed. There are, of course, special cases, and the most special of all is the *Timaeus*, which Plato himself describes as being only probable. But in the *Timaeus*, we have a way of seeing how notions from the popular culture can be combined with Plato's intellectual and artistic imagination to create a great work of art about the body – the dialogue itself – which is both plausible and transporting.[30]

Thus, in view of the status of anatomical and physiological "facts" in Greek medicine and the dependence of later writers on earlier ones and on some of the norms of popular medical culture, the Hippocratic treatises and texts in natural philosophy can, with caution, be used as interpretive modes for earlier statues, in part because their sources lie in the generations in which the statues were made. The absence of a lively flow of empirical data slows and stiffens all intellectual professions (not only the medical one), but it is precisely this slow stiffness which gives later medical treatises a plausible authority as representatives of an earlier intellectual culture.

It may very well be that Greek artists were as slow and as inflexible in relation to anatomical and physiological "facts" as were physicians. Indeed, there is no reason to think that they were more interested in a lively flow of empirical data than were their medical brothers – probably less so, if we place artists in a low position within their contemporary intellectual culture, and in any case, differently so. Whatever the case may have been, for artists as for physicians, most often "facts" were not independent of intellectual "fiction," in the sense that observations and empirical data themselves were subject to theoretical winnowing. I would suggest that the process of selection – specifically, the selection of physical facts that have the air of natural phenomena – was as narrow in sculpture as it was in the Hippocratic treatises and in natural philosophy; "facts" themselves were subject to selective inclusion or rejection. While physicians may have had a system whereby their selection of anatomical and physiological facts could be justified, artists also selected: the contexts of their selections, and instances of some of them, is the subject of chapters 3 and 4.

D: SOUL

Of all the anachronisms which need exclusion in the chronological period covered by this study, that of *psuche*, or soul, is the most prominent, in part because the concept, in a very specific definition, has become an invariable, recognizable, and perennial mental presence for ourselves. It appears to have been so for Greek intellectuals as well. Had the idea of soul not been stabilized in the second half of the fifth century B.C., something as ductile and multivalent would have had to have been invented. Soul is perhaps a difficult and not obvious concept – *une chose pas évidente* – but its stabilization by Socrates, and especially its widespread acceptance in antiquity, simplifies to this day many intellectual and interpretive situations, with a suavity and ductility which should (but for some reason does not) render it quite suspect to intellectuals. The history of the idea of the soul is not at issue here: rather, the forerunners of the idea, or the ragged preliminary definitions before Socrates and Plato put *psuche* into one of its conventional orders, are at issue. The prestige and radiance of the Socratic formula cast – and still casts – many of these forerunners and preliminary definitions into a shade retrospectively. Attempts to explain the earlier variations can seem antiquarian and niggling in comparison with the authority of Socrates' definiton.

Before the middle of the fourth century, grave reservations and strict qualifications must be placed on attributing soul-exhibiting characteristics to works of art. As we have seen, expression of soul – *ta tes psuches erga* – is present in Xenophon's fourth-century account of Socrates' visits to artists' workshops, but what was being discussed in those venues was a well-developed, even pedantically codified, Socratic idea of soul as the immaterial prompter of movements which can have physical manifestations and which can be made evident in artistic representations. In the fifth century, there were plenty of other alternatives to the idea of *psuche*. Among these, we may cite the evolutionary view of human life which is expressed by Aeschylus in his *Prometheus Bound*, especially in Prometheus's speeches "on the arts," with the eventual reward of *dike*, or justice, which seems to be an animating force.[31] Anaxagoras's leading concept, enunciated by him in lectures at Athens in the middle of the fifth century B.C., was that of *nous*, or mind (see below, p. 00), and philosophers who tended toward monistic theories advanced the primacies of various forces or essences. Dramatizations of *isonomia* (roughly, equal application of and equality before a given body of political and municipally based *nomos*) either versus, or parallel to *monarchia* (dominance of one force) were the early respondents to what ultimately would become a widespread acceptance of the idea of soul in medical writing.[32] None of these ideas, it seems to me, can really be represented very fully in works of art. And because the idea of soul was itself a developing concept, the temptation to see it more abundantly than its status in the fifth century can allow must be resisted. The idea of soul in its Socratic manifestation, one which ultimately Aristotle and the writers of medical treatises accepted, defended, elaborated, and learned to prove (both in its physical and in its spiritual manifestations), need not necessarily be excluded from discussions of early classical works of art, but it constitutes, before the mid-fourth century, a conceptual anachronism. Alternatives to it – some of the informing principles of pre-Socratic natural philosophy – are outlined in chapters 3 and 4. These alternatives, which I regard, as I regard the soul, as substantially unrepresentable in works of art, I have cautiously called "animating force" because I think that artists' awareness of such issues may have been a perplexed and questioning, even bemused, one. Certainly their awareness cannot have been as complete as that which existed in the minds of philosophers, nor as specific as modern reconstruction of these matters has become. A more specific designation than "animating force" seems impossible in view of the editing to which the thoughts of pre-Socratic philosophers were subjected by writers in the fourth and subsequent centuries.

These have been methodological considerations; with them, I hope to have clarified some – by no means all – of the ways in which Greek medical and philosophical writing can be brought to bear on statues. The test of them is to be seen in the statues. I have chosen two areas of investigation: first, an area of apparent anomaly among statues of similar style and date and, second, an area of significant changes in the style and iconography of the body, where there are abundant comparisons to be had and made. I begin with an instance of apparent stylistic anomaly in chapter 3. Chapter 4 is about changes in stance (*contrapposto*) and facial expression in male nudes of the Severe style with respect to earlier kouroi. It also defines some of the meanings of *contrapposto* and of facial expression in early classical sculpture.

CHAPTER THREE

Early Classical Statues

Because early classical statues are few in number and even copies of them relatively meagre, it may seem unusual in this discussion to include the statue called the Omphalos Apollo (plates 1–2), particularly since it is used in association with a widely different and original work in relief, the funerary stele of a girl from Paros (plate 3). The Omphalos Apollo is a marble copy of a bronze original of about 480 B.C. Therefore, because it is the kind of copy in which the position of the arms, at the very least, could have been different from the original, why is it included in this discussion? I do so because the copy in question and other versions close to it, such as the Apollo Choiseul-Gouffier, seem to be predicated on an intentional attempt to reproduce, as faithfully and consistently as possible, the style and characteristics of the original – to make a very convincing reproduction of a statue well understood, by the later sculptor and patron, to be an old one. The difference in medium (marble rather than bronze) is obvious, and differences of surface treatment were inevitable. Still, both the Omphalos Apollo and the Apollo Choiseul-Gouffier exhibit old-fashioned proportions, certain peculiarities of stance, and – most important – blood vessels. All of these characteristics are specific to the date and style of the originals and constituted, presumably, the appeal they had for later sculptors and patrons. Whatever the date of the copies (fourth century, Hellenistic, or Roman), their sculptors understood well enough what the characteristics of the original had been. They reproduced them – proportions, stance, and blood vessels – in their copies because these features were integral to the original. Artist-copyists, as well as their patrons, had enough antiquarian intelligence to recognize the importance of these features in the original they were reproducing.

A second reason to include the Omphalos Apollo is that its bronze tionship of the two figures. The descriptive anatomy of the Riace warriors brings them close together in terms of the technical construction of their bodies.

Another contribution, also technical in nature, does the same. The photogrammetric diagrams of the Riace warriors, made and analysed by C. Sena, give an accurate topographical image of the statues, projected like a map with contour lines. These serve to define the structure of the statues' surfaces from all four sides. In consequence, these diagrams clearly distinguish between superficial differences and actual similarities: the differences, due to slight differences of stance, are even more clearly seen than the anatomical description could convey, and conversely, similarities are immediately apparent. As I read them, the topography of the "still" parts of both statues (as opposed to "moving" elements such as arms, necks, and heads) exhibits a quite remarkable similarity. The contours of the upper torsos from the nipples through the shoulders and deltoids, of the areas from the nipples through the knees on the sides of the statues, and of the fleshy parts of both backs from the shoulders through the buttocks were planned, it seems to me, by artists who were close enough to each other to share the same conceptions of physical topography, both in general and in detail. Differences there are, to be sure, but with resepect to anatomy and surface contours, the similarities between the two statues are obvious on the basis of the photogrammetric representations. It must be said that Sena's photogrammetric images of the Riace warriors are among the first such images of Greek statues ever made. Other statues represented in photogrammetic formula might exhibit a similar kind of surface, and even human beings might show a similar topography. However, my instinct tells me otherwise: I am pretty sure that a photogrammetric diagram of the topography of other fifth-century works in similar stances would reveal quite different structures from those of the statues in question. The technique could be developed in order to objectify stylistic evaluation of Greek sculpture, but its results so far are revealing: the photogrammetry of the Riace warriors reveals a striking similarity between them.

Bronze statues of this and other periods do not come all of a piece, and in this instance, as with descriptive anatomy and photogrammetry, both study of the techniques of bronze sculpture and chemical analyses of metals can be crucial to determining issues of date and relationship. In the case of the Riace statues, Warrior B's right arm (from just below the ball of the shoulder; plate 7), right hand, and left forearm (with the mounting for the shield) have a different metallic composition from the rest of the body, higher in lead content and lower in tin. This fact has been advanced to support a later date for the right arm and hand

and the left forearm: E. Formigli, who first discovered the differences in metallic composition in Warrior B, suggested that they might have been Hellenistic repairs, and A. di Vita even proposed that they were Roman. These suggestions were made, it seems to me, in defiance of the visual evidence. As far as I can see, Warrior B exhibits no stylistic inconsistencies or awkwardnesses between his body, feet, and head, on the one hand, and the arms and hands, on the other, which would indicate different dates for them. Technically, of course, like other bronze statues, both Riace warriors were cast in an initial large piece from the neck through the back halves of the feet, and the arms, hands, heads, front feet, and other details were cast separately and added. Thus, differences in metallic composition among the various parts (and from one statue to another) are to be expected. In the case of the percentage of tin relative to copper, variances of more than 10 per cent are commonly found and were found in Warrior B, even in different parts of the initial large piece poured first. Thus the metallic composition, including the higher lead content in Warrior B's arms and hands, does not seem a decisive factor in any argument that they are of a later, or much later, date. Mattusch has sensibly proposed some alternatives to the conclusion that differences of metallic composition denote wide chronological differences, noting among other things that the amount of molten metal for any given pour may have affected its composition. I would add that anyone who has read Benvenuto Cellini's account of the pots, pans, and other objects which he threw into the crucible to improve the flux of the molten metal during the pour of his Perseus in 1554 will realize that ad hoc activity in the atelier is at least as important as consistent following of tested receipes. In any case, the claim by Formigli that the arms are of Hellenistic date seems arbitrary in view of the other published work which he cites.

That said, it may still be that Warrior B's arms were at some time broken off and soldered back on or, at the very most, that they were indeed replaced sometime in antiquity. Whatever the case may have been, what happened to his arms both makes a difference and does not. What is clear is that, whether or not the arms are reapplied originals or later substitutions, the artists involved were concerned enough with the statue's physical authenticity to depict the blood vessels of the upper arms and forearms in a manner compatible with Warrior A and with other statues of the early classical period. In other words, whatever happened to Warrior B's arms, they were worked over by an artist, either a near contemporary or a later one, who recognized an essential feature – the blood vessels – and made it his business to put them in. It can be noted that the same recognition of how crucial the blood vessels were was made by the copyist who created the Omphalos Apollo: he did not leave out something which was essential to the statue, even though he might have been working at a time when veins were no longer commonly represented. Whether this was due to slavish imitation or to genuine historical understanding by the later copyist ultimately makes no difference to my argument, since the blood vessels present in Warrior B's original arms (and in Warrior A's) are there, even if the arms are additions or substitutions.

These technical considerations about the Omphalos Apollo and the Riace warriors establish the series of sculptures of the early classical period which will be under consideration in this chapter. As we shall see, issues of proportions, stance, and blood vessels bring these statues close together, not primarily on stylistic grounds but more on grounds of intellectual context; in turn, it is this intellectual context which prompts discussion of other statues and reliefs.

A: STANCE AND PROFILE

Early classical statues and reliefs made between about 480 and 450 B.C. exhibit a generalized tendency toward heads smaller in proportion to the length of the body than they had been in the first twenty years of the century.[3] It is in this period that the classical proportions in males of about 1:7 (head to body) were formulated. This tendency in proportions is manifested in many works of the period, with two exceptions. In the Omphalos Apollo (plates 1–2) and types derived from it, the head is smaller than the norm, in a proportion of about 1:7½ with respect the length of the body.[4] In contrast, in the funerary stele from Paros in New York (plate 3), depicting a girl with her pet doves, the head is remarkably large in proportion to the body, representing a unit of one to a body length of about five.[5] The anomaly between the proportions of the two figures has been noted, even though their stylistic similarities and proximity in date within the early classical period are not in doubt; their similarities derive from the effect of metallic linear detail in the hair contrasted with the smooth fullness of the flesh, a contrast to which bronze, capable of both smooth treatment and linear cutting with a chisel, lends itself (the original of the Omphalos Apollo was in bronze).[6] I would like to suggest at least three other similarities with respect to anatomy and physiological function between these two works, which are otherwise so different with reference to the sex of the figures shown, the medium of execution (relief and sculpture in the round), the findspot, and so on. The similarities have to do exclusively with certain physical characteristics that both figures exhibit.

The first similarity between them is that both incline their heads forward and down while moving their elbows back and tensing their shoul-

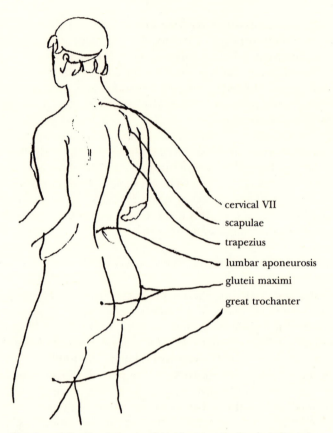

cervical VII

scapulae

trapezius

lumbar aponeurosis

gluteii maximi

great trochanter

Figure 1. Sketches of the Omphalos Apollo with anatomical parts indicated.

ders. The second is that they are among the first statues in the fifth century to exhibit a characteristic which became common later on: a sway-backed silhouette with great prominence and extrusion of buttocks (see section B below). The third similarity is less obvious visually but is very important for other reasons: both figures exhibit respiratory processes (see sections B and C below).

In the case of the girl's head in the stele from Paros, the position is obvious: the face in profile inclines forward toward the bird's beak, and the posterior silhouette of the shoulders, connected under the drapery with the curve of the buttocks where the peplos parts, indicates that the elbow is held well back of the curving line of the back, even though the wrist and hand cradle the dove on her breast. The girl is raising and tensing her shoulders; her peplos hangs straight down, off the ball of the shoulder joint. The back of the buttocks appears where the peplos opens, but the legs themselves are not seen, and the physical impres-

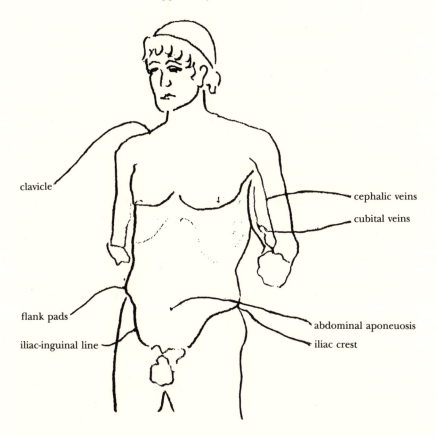

clavicle

cephalic veins

cubital veins

flank pads

abdominal aponeuosis

iliac-inguinal line

iliac crest

sion is one of great prominence of buttocks, in part because the figure, like the Omphalos Apollo, has the sway-backed or S-shaped dorsal curve typical of later figures and quite uncommon earlier. The buttocks are extruded upwards, their profile separated from the legs. The line of the right leg is marked by the drapery, which is held taut because it has perhaps gotten caught in the sandal (the soles of the sandals are shown, but the straps over the instep would have been painted on the feet).

The same elements are easier to see, of course, in the Omphalos Apollo (plates 1–2 and figure 1). In this statue, the stance is conveyed at the expense of anatomical correctness. The forward and downward inclination of the head and neck is shown without the consequent appearance of the first thoracic vertebrae (the vertebra prominens, cervical VII). Instead, the area where the vertebrae should appear is emphatically shown, namely, the upper part of the tendinous floor of the trapezius, interpreted as a deep lozenge-shaped rift between the trapezius muscles and the scapulae (figure 1). This lozenge-shaped depression in the upper back is repeated in larger form lower down to express the area of the lumbar aponeurosis, or flat of the back, and because it is very deeply set with the respect to the lateral muscles, it has the visual effect of separating the buttocks in a marked way. Indeed, the glutei maximi in the Omphalos Apollo are separated and set in different positions to a much more marked degree than those of the Kritios boy a few years before.[7] The asymmetry of the buttocks is indispensible to the *contrapposto* pose, of course, and in the Omphalos Apollo their asymmetry achieved developed form.

In addition, since the depression of the great trochanter of the outer thigh is interpreted as rising into the gluteus medius on the back, the effect of upward thrust of the buttocks and of their emphatic furrow at the intersection with the legs indicates that the sculptor, like the sculptor of the Paros stele, thought of the buttocks as quite distinctly different in shape, musculature, and plane from the legs. If one compares these elements in the Omphalos Apollo with the same ones in the Kritios boy, it is clear from the comparison, and also from comparison with all other standing male nudes of the second half of the sixth century, that the sway-backed silhouette, buttocks, gluteal folds and furrows, and the separation of the buttocks from the legs are anatomically much more emphatic in the Omphalos Apollo than they had previously been, with some exceptions in the seventh and very early sixth centuries (Mantiklos figure; possibly Kleobis and Biton).[8] Kouroi were sharply articulated or softly sculpted as manifestations of a regional tradition or an artist's individual style, but the separation of surface and plane among their parts had never been as emphatically treated as it was in the Omphalos Apollo.

The original of the Omphalos Apollo represented the early moments of the Severe style around 480 B.C. The Riace warriors stand at the end of it or at the very beginning of the high classical period, around 460–450 B.C. Warrior B has sometimes been dated later than his mate, but as indicated above, I am convinced, from evidence of bodily characteristics they exhibit, that the warriors are very close to each other in date and workmanship (see p. oo and n. oo).

Both Riace warriors (plates 5–9) have inclined necks and slightly tilting heads with sway-backed silhouettes similar to the Severe style figures. While their upper backs are differently structured from that of the Omphalos Apollo, their lower backs have sacrospinalis muscles which swell prominently and descend steeply into the sacral triangle to emphasize the gluteal fold in the same way. In the Riace statues, the deep gluteal furrows and the artificial extension of the depression of the great trochanter into the glutei medii are very similar to the same features in the Omphalos Apollo.

From this evidence, it is with statues of the early classical period about 480 B.C., of which the Omphalos Apollo (or rather the original of it) is an example, that the anatomical norm for male figures was formulated with respect to sway-backed stance, deep lower back, and separation of buttocks from each other and from the legs, with upward extrusion and prominence. The proportions (head to body = c. 1:7½) of the Omphalos Apollo were not reused later in the fifth century, but the relationship of many of his internal parts endured and was applied to later statues. His characteristics appear, in profile but in the same relationship, in the figure of the girl from Paros and even more prominently in another profile figure, that of the young man on a funerary stele from Nisyros (plate 12). This figure's high-waisted, long body and small head are the proportional equivalents of the Omphalos Apollo, even though the fullness of his body and his profile make him almost the girl's elder brother.[9]

All these figures – the Paros girl, the Omphalos Apollo, and the Riace warriors – lift their arms upward and move their elbows back behind the dorsal silhouette. They do so to a degree much greater than all earlier kouroi, and greater, too, than certain figures closer to them in date (c. 530–480 B.C.), such as the Piraeus Apollo, Aristodikos, and the Kritios boy.[10] In these last statues, the elbows retreat, but certainly not as far back as they do in the Omphalos and Riace figures. In late-sixth-century figures, the detachment of the hands from the thighs *did* coincide with a little greater flexion backward at the elbows. While the "elbows back" stance might have been suggested from earlier figures, the sculptors of the Severe style actually invented a new bodily position in Greek physical representation, because "elbows back" was accompanied by a change in the shoulders. The Omphalos Apollo, the Riace warriors, the *Doryphoros* of Polykleitos (what can be told from the copies), and especially the forward-facing male nudes in the pediments of the temple of Zeus at Olympia all have tensed, raised shoulders, giving a square frontal silhouette to the upper body.[11] In contrast, most earlier kouroi, with a very few possible exceptions (Kleobis and Biton much earlier and Aristodikos around 500 B.C.), are slack shouldered. Despite stylistic and dating differences and/or varieties of provenance and medium, what is emphatic in the anatomy of kouroi throughout the sixth century and up to about 480 B.C. is the long, relaxed silhouette of the trapezius and its smooth flow into the neck (in the sterno-mastoid area). The effect is achieved in long-haired, long-necked kouroi by masking the sharp change of direction with a fall of hair uniting head and shoulders and in short-haired, short-necked kouroi by unduly widening the neck and/or softening the line of the trapezius and sternomastoid curve.

In contrast to the kouroi, male nudes of the early classical period and many in the high classical period have tense, high shoulders. The deltoids are raised at the sides. On the back, the scapulae and the infraspinatus muscles are almost always merged as kidney-shaped bulges instead of the soft separate ovals of late archaic statues; this adds mass to the upper back, giving an effect of tension. On the front, there is an acute angle between the horizontal of the clavicle and the silhouette of the trapezius, an angle much more acute than the more oblique clavicle-trapezius intersection of earlier statues, including Aristodikos and the Kritios boy. In archaic figures, the conception of the shoulders had been of a swanning upward flow of the silhouette toward the neck and a forward, slack stance in the shoulders. With the Omphalos Apollo and after him, throughout much of the fifth century, the usual stance was one of tension and lift in arms and shoulders, with an emphasis, not on continuity of surface, but on marked separation of parts and functions in a very well developed, indeed athletically conditioned, physique. It is such physiques showing sharp definition of parts that the author of *Physiognomics* approved of because they were highly readable (81ob.35–811a.5). Definition and separation of parts is the descriptive method of medical treatises as well; the author of *On Joints* described the functional movement and progression of bodies in detail, noting in his analysis, the subdivisions of function and specialized form of each part (*On Joints* 1.18–32; 8.59–63; 58.84–90).[12] He often warned his fellow-physicians about how difficult, but how necessary, it was to get a patient with a dislocation or fracture to relax his muscles. In the fifth century, the effect of tense, raised shoulders with contraction of the deltoids gave the effect of pectoral breathing, an effect which was intentional, as I will show in section B. In addition, the raised shoulders naturally threw the upper arms into supine position, for reasons outlined in section C.

Thus, despite differences in medium and despite the fact that the figures depicted are of different sexes and that one of them is a Roman copy, the stele from Paros and the Omphalos Apollo are similar in at least two respects – the stance of their heads and elbows and the tension of their shoulders – and also in their sway-backed, prominently buttocked silhouettes. In fact, it is precisely these characteristics which mark the difference between them and earlier figures; it is the same characteristics that makes them similar to each other and to other figures of the fifth century. The strong definition of parts and the effect of tension came to be quite widely applied by various sculptors of the classical period to situations quite different from the specific four statues we have been looking at.

B: RESPIRATION

With the third similarity between the Omphalos Apollo and the girl from Paros (plates 1–3), that of inhalation in both figures, the physiological function is quite differently depicted. The girl is doing one of two things (neither much approved of by most parents). Either she is nuzzling her pet or else she has placed a seed, which could have been painted in, between her lips, and she is enjoying the bird's pecking it out – Aristotelian writers say that the lips are the most ticklish part of the body, more so than the armpits (*Problems* 965a.18–19). If she is nuzzling the dove, her lips are firmly closed. If she has a seed between her lips, she is holding it by tensing her lips and breathing through her nostrils. In either case, the respiratory function of inhalation or "about to inhale" through her nose is necessary.

There is another indication of her breathing in the drapery. In cradling the dove, the girl has also lifted the hem of the *apoptygma* (overhang) of her peplos. This reveals that she has lost the *zone*, or belt, which both closed the peplos at the sides and allowed adjustment of its length. The peplos has swung open, revealing her buttocks and back. Peploi, secured by pins at the shoulders, were let out a little long in front and back, and because the cloth was slack at the wearer's halter and yoke, the garment would open at the sides and fall to the ground if not secured by a belt. The length of a peplos at the feet was adjusted by blousing the material above the belt, which could be either over the *apoptygma* or beneath it at the level of the hips and lower abdomen. In the stele, this is exactly what has happened. The *apoptygma* in the front has been lifted to show that inhalation, which swells the abdomen ([Aristotle] *Problems* 964a.39–965b.4), has also broken or unknotted the *zone* (which could have been painted falling). The blousing at the level of the belt has fallen out, and the lower hem has slid down and folded over the feet in front. (Correctly belted, it should "break" over the instep like men's trousers in the manner that Jeeves insisted upon for his well-dressed employer, Bertie Wooster).[13] Behind her foot, the peplos has fallen to the ground and drags behind the heel; the girl would trip if she moved forward. There are other instances of unbelted peploi, also on funerary stelai, but this is the first instance, to my knowledge, of action, stance, and drapery combining to indicate inhalation in a figure.[14] The small drama of the drapery and the broken or unknotted belt clearly indicate the physiology of respiration, and although her mouth is not open, the girl from Paros can in other ways be related stylistically to open-mouthed figures at Olympia. Later on, the Riace warriors are both open-mouthed and inhaling, as we shall see.

More difficult is the interpretation of what inhalation meant in the Paros stele. The temptation is to apply a complex and resolutely esoteric, but more or less contemporary, interpretation to the physiological action, namely the Pneumatic theory, which Aristotle describes in order to refute. This theory, according to which *pneuma*, or breath (air), in the world was either the same thing as, or else a little thicker than, the Pneumatic soul, or animate force, is first datable to the 540s because it was propounded by Anaximenes of Miletus (fl. 546 B.C.). The Pneumatic theory of the soul reappeared in the encyclopedic book by Anaxagoras of Clazomenae (fl. 460–430 B.C.) and later in the thought of Diogenes of Apollonia and Democritus of Abdera early in the second half of the fifth century (Aristotle *On the Soul* 403b.30–404a.25, 410b.28–30; *On Respiration* 471b.30–472b.5).[15] It should be pointed out that, as reported by Aristotle, the Pneumatic soul is a thing which occupies space and which has a time- and space-bound trajectory; we are still far from the Socratic soul.

The Pneumatic theory of the soul was thus verifiably current around the time that the girl from Paros was made; it seems to have been an idea of long-standing authority, because it received important elaborations and uses subsequent to its first appearance in the thought of Anaximenes. Put simply, a Pneumatic interpretation of her action could be read as follows: the soul (or its Pneumatic equivalent), being itself air or thin air, remains in the body by virtue of the inhaled outer air (thicker or heavier) not letting it be expelled. The notion is that, at all times in a living creature, there must be some outer air inside the body to counteract the outer air's external pressure on the body. When respiration stops, the heavier outer air or the weight of the body itself presses the soul-like *pneuma* outward. If we assume that the doves in this stele represent either the soul-like *pneuma* or vehicles for the taking away of it and if we assume that this is the girl's last breath, one deep enough to have broken her belt, then what we are witnessing is a Pneumatic scene, one in which the genre image is elaborated, as genre images can be, into a scene of greater significance, in this case an account of the departure of the *pneuma* from the body. Such an account might well have had a genuine place in Pneumatic physiology.

There are difficulties in this interpretation. In the first place, in strictly argued Pneumatic physiology, if we are to believe Aristotle's and others' accounts of it, the soul-like *pneuma* shared with air its invisibility and continuous self-generated motion.[16] For that reason, it needed neither an attribute nor a vehicle (in either case the doves – and why two doves?). And if we assume that the patron and the sculptor, who would not have been strictly arguing Pneumatic philosophers, wished nevertheless to depict such a situation, we would have to see it in other appropriate *semeia* in the work itself or in other works. As it happens, in these years, Pindar used the removal of the belt (not its breaking) as a metaphor for childbirth (*Olympian* 4.39–40), and it is used as a metaphor for marriage and sexual intercourse in the *Odyssey* (2.245), but it is not used as a metaphor for death, and it does not have the value that "ungirt" does in Shakespeare. The actual breaking of the *zone* does not appear in other stelai, though beltless peplophoroi do, but without specific attributes or actions of death. Metaphorically, the seed or grain (*sitos*) that may be painted between the girl's lips can mean "civilized men" as opposed to savages (Hesiod *Works and Days* 146), but the reference seems too generalized. [17] I can find no instance of tripping (over the hem of the peplos) to refer to death, though I believe that the girl is standing still, left foot forward, with the weight on the right leg. In fact, she is one of the first figures to exhibit *contrapposto*. The stance of the legs and feet themselves can have an iconographic meaning, but in quite another context (see chapter 4). Finally, the contemporary metope of the Girdle of the Amazon, an adventure of Heracles on the temple of Zeus at Olympia, does not seem to me to have useful meanings for any interpretation of the stele. This being the case, it seems better to limit the interpretation of the girl's action to one of inhalation (if anything, a sign of life) and to see the stele as depicting a genre scene, even at the risk of being too positivistic. There is, however, an important extension to the meaning of inhalation, as we shall see in section C.

Statues earlier than the Omphalos Apollo and the Riace warriors may or may not be inhaling, but even if they were, inhalation was not shown to the same degree of anatomical precision with which it is shown in the girl from Paros. In the Omphalos Apollo and especially in the Riace warriors (plates 5–9), the sculptors redesigned the anatomy of the abdomen, flank pads, and iliac furrow with a view to describing the physiological effect of inhalation.

The visual conjunction of these three elements – abdomen, flank pads, and iliac furrow – was effected by the redesigning of what I call the "iliac-inguinal line." This feature is mainly artistic, only partially anatomical. The iliac-inguinal line in classical statues is the line or shape defined by the swelling flesh above the iliac crest (crista iliaca) in the area of the flank pads; the line changes direction over the iliac spine (spina iliaca anterior superior) and descends along a curving line (that of a radically redesigned inguinal ligament) to the genitals. Ordinarily, the whole shape from the iliac crest to the genitals is shown in statues as a furrow between two planes of flesh, as if the abdomen were a bag pressing over an armature covering the upper legs. Anatomically, what is being represented is the abdominal aponeurosis of tendons in front and, to the side, the outlines of the iliac crest and iliac spine (which in statues have balls of muscle or fat applied to them). The inguinal ligament is, anatomically, straight and not connected to the iliac spine directly; in statues, it curves and has a fleshy, rather than a thinned, appearance. The design of the iliac-inguinal line as a curving furrow was an artistic one, not corresponding to palpable anatomical features.

All kouroi in the sixth century and most later Greek male nudes exhibit this well-known emphatic marking of the iliac-inguinal line. In kouroi, it is represented sometimes as a groove, sometimes as a narrow, sausage-like roll, or sometimes as a shadow between two curving surfaces.[18] The iliac-inguinal line can assume quite different shapes, at times straight, in other kouroi curving in different ways, but what was stabilized after the early classical figures is the shape that it had in the copies of the *Doryphoros* of Polykleitos, namely, a steeply descending lower V with curving upper horns. Inside and above it, the whole abdomen and the flank pads billow and swell outward and over the furrow, whose tough line crisply separates the hips and legs from the torso. The effect is one of inflation in the lower abdomen, and the swelling flank pads sometimes merge with the glutei medii at the back, as if an underlying respiratory organ were expanding the whole frontal lower torso.

This treatment became the norm for male nudes through Hellenistic and into Roman times, with only minor variations. Since the figures are mostly quite sway-backed, the effect of forward swell in the abdomen was visually accentuated to a marked degree when the statues are viewed in profile. The Kritios boy had this effect of swelling abdomen, but to a much lesser degree than the Omphalos Apollo, and earlier statues are characterized by flat abdominal profiles.[19]

Another element of the torso which the sculptors redesigned in the Omphalos Apollo, and which also appears in the Riace warriors, is the contrast between the swelling flank pads and the ribs. The contrast is emphasized to show inhalation, like the new emphasis on the swelling abdomen and the new shape of the iliac-inguinal line. The flank pads are called *laparai* in Greek (also meaning sausages), and they have a potential for physiognomic meaning. However, what is obvious in these statues is that the thickness of the flank pad is intended to contrast with the thinning of the skin over the ribs above. The Omphalos Apollo is proudly showing us five of his ribs on each side, more than any kouros ever did, and the Riace warriors, although they have fewer ribs (only four) and the ones they have are more softly defined and digitated, nevertheless have an emphatic curving shape in the ribcage, and the line of the thorax and diaphragm is extremely prominent. Upon inhalation, of course, the lower abdomen and the flank pads swell forward, but the ribs rise upward and outward and can be counted through the skin.[20] An emphatic flank pad – ribs contrast is evident, and this contrast is what the sculptor included in the new design of the torso.

By the end of the fifth century, this external effect of the mechanism of respiration was well known and had been fully described medically (Plato *Timaeus* 78c; Aristotle *On Respiration* 480a.16–480b.12).[21] Moreover, when the Hippocratic discourse *On Breaths* was written, in the first half of the fourth century, the contrast among the different parts of the torso below the midriff was dramatically emphasized verbally – *laparai*, hypochondrium (the area between diaphragm and navel), ribs, and lower abdomen – in the same way that the flank pads – ribs contrast was dramatized by the sculptors (*On Breaths* 9).[22]

Inflation of the abdomen and the flank pad – ribs contrast are the main signs of inhalation in these statues, but there are other indicators as well. The Omphalos Apollo's mouth was shut, but that of the girl from Paros, though not open, had tension at the lips; there were open-mouthed figures at Olympia, and the Riace warriors and the *Doryphoros* are also open-mouthed. The open mouths of these statues are the equivalent of Aristotle's refutation of the physiology of respiration advanced by Empedocles (fl. 450 B.C.). Empedocles' theory of respiration was made on analogy with the *klepsydra*, or water-clock, and he thought that only one opening was the primary one for human breathing, that of the nostrils (Aristotle *On Respiration* 473a.15–474a.24).[23] Aristotle's refutation of Empedocles' idea is detailed, and he insisted, against what seems to have been an enduring notion, that breathing is equally effective through either the nostrils or the mouth. Plato had already said so (*Timaeus* 79c.2) and had agreed with Aristotle on the fact that inhalation inflates the abdomen (*Timaeus* 78c–d; cf. [Aristotle] *Problems* 964a.39–965b.4), though for slightly different but highly significant reasons, namely, Plato believed that there was some direct connection through the windpipe with a lung-like apparatus in the abdomen (in the inguinal area below the hypochondrium and navel, not just with the lungs in the upper torso). Plato's analogy was that of wicker baskets or fish traps set into a larger one (the body itself) and bobbing up and down inside it (cf. *The Sacred Disease* 10). He said this because, like Empedocles, he regarded respiration as a nutritive function for the body and the soul (for which reason, air must reach well down into the body cavity), whereas Aristotle, who considered respiration to be refrigerative (air is cold and dry), used the analogy of the bellows to explain inguinal inflation: collapsed when blowing out, inflated when drawing air in, and air went to the lungs exclusively. The multiplication of analogies is confusing, but the point is that by the mid-fifth century and throughout the fourth, the physiology of breathing through the mouth was an issue of great importance in physiological speculation, and also where air went in the body, how it got there, and what it did (cf. *On Nutriment* 30). The tension of the shoulders and the open mouths of the fifth-century figures are emblems, or *semeia*, of their respiration when taken with their swelling abdomens, the new depth and shape of the iliac-inguinal line, and the flank pad – ribs contrast.

In visual terms, the redesigning of the abdomen by sculptors in the early classical period did what writers on physique also did, namely, establish correspondences among the parts of the body on the basis of anatomical structure and physiological function.[24] The sculptors, in connecting faces, open mouths, shoulders, and abdomens in their figures, made the same correspondence among these parts that was vigorously and crisply described by physicians and philosophers. Moreover, it is no accident that they chose these particular correspondences to make because, as we shall see, Aristotle speaks both about the scientific basis and about popular beliefs and medical practices concerning a "nether face" or a "nether head" below the navel, in the precise area of those features which the sculptors redesigned (see chapter 4). In addition, when we come to consider the stance, setting, and character of the eyes in the archaic and classical periods, we will have to discuss the new shape of the buttocks, because eyes and buttocks had a curious, old, and popular interconnection in Greek physiological thinking (see p. 88).

It remains to be seen what the iconography of inhalation is in the Omphalos Apollo and the Riace warriors. We have seen the extreme difficulties in applying the theories of Pneumatic activity and physiology to the bodily action of the girl on the stele from Paros, even though the stele and that idea of the soul as *pneuma* were more or less contemporaneous with her. At the risk of repeating myself, let me recapitulate the Greek medical theories of respiration. Natural philosophers by the fourth century had many and various views on the topic: Plato thought that respiration was a nutritive function and that it fed, in some way, the nutritive part of the soul, whereas Aristotle was at pains to convince his students that the effect of air in the body reinforced what the brain also did, namely, to refrigerate it. Earlier, by the late fifth century, physicians in the Hippocratic corpus had developed their own ideas about respiration, but speaking in very general terms, what the physicians discovered clinically, and ultimately what they could not agree upon interpretively, was that respiration, movement, exercise, and physiognomic signs were interconnected and that all these were connected in various ways with the veins and pulses in the body.[25] Our alternatives of interpretation, that is, respiration as Pneumatic activity, respiration as nutritive function, or respiration as refrigerative effect, cannot properly proceed without considering the veins in the body. Observation of the veins and auscultation of the thorax in the fifth century allowed physicians to hear and feel what they listen for and feel today, namely, the pulse, the rhythm of breath, and the dynamic thudding of the heart (the last two they did not distinguish; cf. *On the Heart* 8).

C: VEINS AND FLEXION

As it happens, the Omphalos Apollo and the Riace warriors are, to my knowledge, among the first standing Greek statues to have superficial veins systematically and consistently shown in their torsos, arms, hands, and feet, with greatly detailed emphasis by their sculptors (plates 1, 5–9). In this they follow a slightly earlier trend: Pliny mentions that the sculptor Pythagoras of Rhegium, who worked in Italy and at Olympia in the first quarter of the fifth century, was the first to depict veins and sinews as well as carefully represented hair (*Natural History* 34.59).

The history of veins on statues in the classical period is short. In general, veins no longer appear on statues by the beginning of the fourth century B.C., though they do reappear on statues at Tegea and also in Hellenistic times.[26] The medical reasons for the later disappearance and the subsequent reappearance of the superficial veins in statues cannot be discussed here; I am concerned only with the appearance of veins in early classical figures and in the Riace warriors. To be sure, as a general phenomenon, anatomical features can go in and out of fashion in statues quite as quickly as clothing styles do on people, and with the same unpredictability and difficulties of interpretation. However, I am not disposed to accept the sudden appearance of veins on male bodies in the fifth century as a mere stylistic quirk, because *what veins do* was a major intellectual and clinical question, and when we hear about the problem in the Hippocratic corpus, it is plain that it was a complex, long-standing issue.[27] Blood vessels were importantly connected with the soul in its early definitions or with other animating forces. Aristotle lists several late-sixth-and fifth-century philosophers who, like Plato, the Pneumatists, and Critias (who thought that soul was blood), used various analyses of the anatomy and/or physiology of the veins to demonstrate the effect of animating forces on the body (*On the Soul* 403b.20–405b.10).

The similarity of the Omphalos Apollo and the girl from Paros on the basis of their stylistic affinities and the similarity of stance (heads, arms, and shoulders), distribution of parts (sway-back and prominence of buttocks), and physiological function (inhalation) brought them closer together than the apparent dissimilarity of their external proportions and their other differences would suggest. But the issue of blood vessels reminds us that the girl from Paros (plate 3) is different from the Omphalos Apollo in another respect: she has no veins in her arms or hands. As far as I am aware, no Greek female figure has superficial veins, either on reliefs where their male companions exhibit them prominently, for example, in the east side of the Parthenon frieze, where the stocky elders who are marshalling the maidens have emphatic hand and arm veins and the maidens none at all, or in single statues of women in any period of Greek art when male figures had veins (or, for that matter, when they did not).[28] The only exceptions are Hellenistic statues of old women, whose hand and arm veins are sometimes visible because the body was emaciated with age (cf. Aristotle *History of Animals* 511b.20). Of course, superficial veins are easier to see in men than in women, because women have a distribution of subcutaneous tissues different from that of men. But as we shall see, Greek anatomical and physiological speculation virtually precluded women from having superficial veins anyway.

When Aristotle outlined the difficulties of describing the physiology of blood vessels, he summed up the clinical problems which all Greek physicians had, namely, that looking at the veins of freshly killed animals was not much help in understanding what vessels do and whence they come. This is because of the venous collapse and arterial evacuation which occurs at death. In addition, if the physician had based his interpretation on observation of emaciated patients, he could only observe the superficial anatomy of veins (*History of Animals* 511.b11–22, 513a.14 and 20). The clinical conditions for carrying out observations probably led to the major mistake made in Greek medicine about blood vessels: the assumption that some blood vessels contained air, others only blood, or that some or all vessels contained a combination of the two or both air and blood with the addition of other elements.[29] This mistake – that there was air in the blood vessels – resulted, as I have said, from the arterial evacuation of the blood vessels in animals killed for clinical or sacrificial purposes. Thus veins were interpreted as having different origins in the body. Some of these interpretations can be dated. By the late fifth century and in the first half of the fourth, the two major current notions were that the source of blood vessels was in the brain only or in both the brain and heart. By the mid-fourth century, the Hippocratic tendency to revise and clarify the ancient humoral theory, combined with the physicians' desire to locate the soul in the body very accurately, prompted placing the source of the vessels lower down, either in the heart only or in the heart and liver (the better to dramatize the seats of bile, opposing the liver, in the etiology of diseases; cf. *Nutriment* 31). Plato in the *Timaeus* (70b–d) stated that the heart is the knot and source of blood vessels, which also contained air. A little later, Aristotle placed the origin of the vessels (blood only) in the heart exclusively, and he both summed up earlier thinking and settled the issue, medically speaking, for most later thinking. He also modified an older idea, namely, that the soul was *in* the heart, by saying that the soul was "near" the heart.[30] Aristotle could have learned about the older ideas regarding the location of the soul in such Hippocratic treatises as *On the Heart*, where the soul was said to reside in the left ventricle (*History of Animals* 511b ff.; *Parts of Animals* 666a.25–35; cf. *On the Heart* 10).

Thus, insofar as we can trust Aristotle's account, Greek physicians' alternatives for the locations of the source of blood and blood vessels were brain, or brain and heart, or heart and liver, or heart only. The choices were generally made on what the physicians thought the originating organs did. Greek physicians also had a sense that the blood is impelled through the veins in some way – and air as well, if they thought that air was in the veins; this is implied in *On Fractures*, where the lower arm must be raised in a wrapped splint to inhibit blood flow impelled from somewhere above the elbow (*On Fractures* 4.19). These are, in general, the ways in which the blood and blood vessels were understood, and although there are some variations in the fifth century and later, the principles were much the same (cf. Aristotle *History of Animals* 511b.11–513a.14; Diogenes of Apollonia, in Simplicius *Physica* 153.13).

Superficial veins are most visible at the points of flexion in the human body; both physicians and sculptors recognized this. In the Omphalos Apollo and in the Riace warriors (plates 1–2, 5–9), the following superficial veins can be seen, combined with the following points of flexion:

1 In the upper arms, the cephalic veins are particularly prominent and cross well over the armpit into the pectoral muscles of the upper torso. Visually, the sculptors thought of them as connecting the torso with the arms, but they must have had another reason for believing this, because of this peculiarity which all three statues share: at the expense of anatomical accuracy and mechanical possibility, the sculptors positioned the upper arm and elbow in a marked *supine* position (facing out as far as possible) so the biceps and cephalic veins are frontally visible, whereas below the elbows (in both arms in the Omphalos Apollo and in the Riace warriors' right arms), the lower arm and hand are in *prone* positions, with the inner forearm and

palms facing inward. The physical awkwardness of this (it makes for an elbow with more twist in it than elbows have) was masked by the tense-shouldered and elbows-back stance which I have already described, and the intention was to ensure that the cephalic veins in the upper arms would be clearly visible from the front. Supination and pronation of extremities had apparently entered the Hippocratic taxonomy by the end of the fifth century, and the two attitudes were clearly distinguished from each other (*On Joints* and *On Fractures*, passim).[31] The sculptors seem to have been proud of their statues' veins, and they wanted to show them no matter what mechanical improbabilities or impossibilities of stance were involved.

2 In the elbows and lower arms, the join of the cephalic and cubital veins is emphatic, its marked visibility due to the pronation of the elbow. The cubital vein in the Omphalos Apollo and in Riace warrior A ends near where it should, around the base of the biceps, whereas in Riace warrior B it ends higher up, near the middle of the biceps and marking its inner line. In the lower arms of both Riace warriors, the cephalic vein is prominent to the palm at the base of the thumb, and its position is contrasted by the flow of two accessory cephalic veins across the forearm. The emphatic presence of these veins is marked by yet another anatomical deformation, namely, that the lower arm is represented with a distinct and sudden inward and downward bend in the radius bone, at a position up about a third or a quarter of the distance from the wrist to the elbow. This bend gives shapeliness to the lower arm which contrasts with the straight silhouette of the upper arm, and it emphasizes the bifurcation of the veins on the back of the arm.[32] Lower down, the cephalic vein swells at the head of the ulna to a marked degree.

3 In the hands of the Riace warriors, the bifurcation of the cephalic vein above the crotch of the thumb is marked, and veins appear below the wrist in conjunction with the dorsal bones and with two or three long, V-shaped swellings intended to represent sinews. The dorsal and digital venous arches are not shown because the general treatment of the hand is as an object with parallel linear articulations overlapped by veins which are themselves running more or less parallel after bifurcating.

4 In the torso of Riace warrior B (plate 9), on the lower left side only, the superficial epigastric veins (tegumenta) appear very prominently just below the lower part of the ribcage and bifurcate near the upper level of the flank pad, one part descending through the iliac-inguinal line into the upper leg for about ten centimetres, the other snaking down toward the penis and disappearing in the inguinal area as the lower abdomen swells outward in inhalation.

5 In the back and legs of all three statues, veins are not shown; the raised areas or grooves which criss-cross the legs seem to be indications of sinewy separation between bone and calf muscles. In the feet of the Riace warriors, the great saphenous vein swells forward very prominently above the malleolus of the tibia (inner ankle bone), crosses it, and descends on the upper and inner plane of the foot to divide, as in the hand near the thumb, above the great toe to connect with the toes individually. In Warrior B, accessory saphenous veins are shown behind the ankle as well, very prominent and full.

This description clarifies which veins the sculptors emphasized, and it gives us a sense of the relative importance of the veins in different parts of the body. Veins in the neck and back were not shown, but those connecting the breast to the arms were very important, even to the extent of showing an extension of the cephalic vein onto the pectorals, where it does not, in fact, appear anatomically. The veins at the points of flexion (armpits, inner elbows, wrists, and ankles) are also prominent, and together with the emphatic flexion of both knees, the sculptors were representing the human anatomical characteristic of opposite flexion of the upper and lower extremities, which Aristotle emphasized as being something only human beings have, in a context which makes clear that human progression and movement are superior to all other animal structures (*Progression of Animals* 712a.1–21). Aristotle may have made much of this characteristic because of the emphasis which it had in Hippocratic descriptions of the joints: all of the treatments for dislocated limbs in *On Joints* and *On Fractures* assume this anatomical progression of parts, and the mechanisms of the machines used to reduce or extend dislocations were designed with it in mind (*Mochlikon*, passim).[33] The sculptors were anxious to show the characteristic, with the result that they used veins to mark the points of flexion at the wrists and ankles. To show the flexion of the elbows in the same manner, they placed the upper arm in prone and the lower arm in supine attitude, thereby giving themselves a broad, forward-facing field on which to show the join of the cephalic and cubital veins.

That this distortion made for a very twisted elbow with too much pronation did not matter to them. The sculptors were not engaged in descriptive anatomy. They were involved in manipulating the body for effectiveness and clarity, and in this respect they were more like bone-setters than physicians. But a quick bone-setter, after all, is more welcome to a patient with a dislocated shoulder than a descriptive anatomist would be; in the same way, a sculptor who is willing to abandon anatomical "truth" in favour of strong, effective measures which produce visual and iconographic clarity is welcome to us.[34]

The marking of the joints with veins thus satisfies one iconographic aspect of physique in statues, that of stressing its uniquely human character (the opposite flexion of the extremities), but there are other physiological ones as well. In the Riace warriors, great emphasis was put on the accessory cephalic veins in the lower arms and the dorsal veins of the hands, interpreted as crossing over from elbow to hand and bifurcating to connect fingers or toes to wrists or ankles respectively. In other words, a lot of blood is in the hands and feet, and the veins are the fullest at the wrist and ankles and most prominent on the dorsal sides of the extremities.

There are two medical and philosophical reasons for this depiction of the veins. The first is an old interpretation of what was, once again, uniquely human about human anatomy, namely, the one proposed by Anaxagoras (fl. 460–430 B.C.) around the time or a little before these statues were made. Anaxagoras thought that it was the possession of hands which made man the most intelligent of all beings (Aristotle *Parts of Animals* 687a.7).[35] This beautiful pre-Socratic notion reappears in Aristotle's equally splendid simile of the hand being like the soul (*On the Soul* 432a.1). His simile is appropriate in this context because he says that the soul's ability to perceive and use sense perceptions is like the hand's ability to touch objects and use tools. Aristotle's language and the simile itself were induced, I believe, by his recollection of an earlier notion, that of Critias of Athens (fl. 430 B.C.), who had proposed it a little after the time that the statues were made. Critias believed that the soul is blood, because sense perception is the primary characteristic of both blood and soul. This notion of what the soul might be was apparently a popular one and commanded widespread acceptance. Critias's statement is an elegant and succinct version of what the writer of *Nature of Man* a few years later cited as being a common and more muddled notion of blood being soul (*On the Soul* 405b.6–7; cf. 404b.8–11 and *Nature of Man* 6.9–11).[36] Aristotle, by the way, was of the same opinion as Critias in relating blood to sense perception, but he thought that the body, not the soul, was blood (*Parts of Animals* 666a.34–666b.1; 668a.4–7, 10–13). Soul, sense perception, and intelligence – the components of humanness – thus had an established and intimate interconnection with hands and blood in the fifth century, and their relationships must have been complex and interesting if we may judge them by the unexpected splendour of Aristotle's similes when he thinks of them.

The second reason for the fullness of the veins in the wrists, ankles, hands, and feet of the Riace statues is that medically, it exhibits the *nutritive* function of blood and air in the physiology of respiration (not Pneumatic activity or refrigerative effect). This idea is one which corresponds closely to the visual emphasis on the veins in the arms of the

Omphalos Apollo and in the arms and hands of the Riace warriors, and the idea was current in the thought of Empedocles a generation before. In turn, Empedocles' physiology of air in the veins was extended into an anatomical description of the blood vessels by the physician who wrote *Nature of Man*, perhaps around 400 B.C. or a little later. Finally, the speaker who delivered the discourse *On Breaths*, a work in circulation by the mid-fourth century, developed a plausible etiology for the notion, even though his own ideas differ in many respects from those of his predecessors.[37]

The idea is as follows: in the vitalism of Empedocles' general system, the four elements (air, earth, fire, and water) mix with Love and Strife to create the human soul (Aristotle, *On the Soul* 404b.10–15). This idea led Empedocles to the notion that the soul – still in a rather palpable, conditional, composite, and pre-Socratic manifestation – is nourished continuously by contact with the four elements and, in the case of air, through both the lungs and the skin, in a manner that Plato regarded as quite plausible as well (cf. *Timaeus* 79c). Empedocles illustrated his notion by analogy to the water-clock, which I have already mentioned in the context of the nostrils and the open mouths of statues of this period.[38] Its elaboration included a physiology of pulses and respiration whereby inhalation filled the veins with blood (the rising of the pulse was the *semeion* of this process), then the blood retreated (exhalation), and air entered some or all the veins transcutaneously through the pores, with the fall of the pulse as the *semeion* of the completion of the process (Aristotle *On Respiration* 473b.2–474a.6; Aristotle does not fully understand Empedocles' physiology because of a mistaken philological derivation). Empedocles noted that this double respiratory process (nasal and transcutaneous) could be registered at the extremities (474a.3–6). In our terms, the diastolic phase of the pulse represented air entering through the pores into the veins, while, at the systolic phase, air was being pushed out again through the skin in equal amount.

The anatomical elaboration of this notion of transcutaneous respiration was well developed, as an idea, by the time of writing of *Nature of Man* some fifty years later (c. 400 B.C.). This treatise has a strong Empedoclean tendency, as shown in its chapters 1–8. The treatise continued (11) with a detailed description of the blood vessels, and when the author came to describe the "fourth pair" (figure 2) he defined them as the visible ("thick") ones, with their source at the brain and eyes, passing invisibly under the neck and collar-bones, then reappearing in the upper arms, elbows, lower arms, wrists, and fingers, and passing *back again upward* to the armpit following the inner part of the upper arm, exactly as they do in the Omphalos Apollo and the Riace

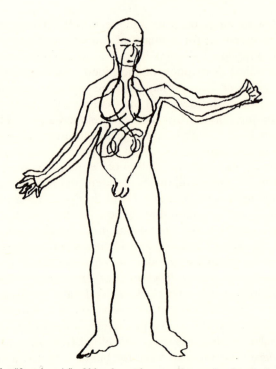

Figure 2. The "fourth pair" of blood vessels according to the description in *Nature of Man*.

warriors (plates 1–2, 5–8).[39] In the case of Warrior B (plate 9), the description of the veins as going back upward again from the hand is particularly appropriate because, in his upper arm, the cubital vein marks almost the entire inner surface of the biceps, as the author of *Nature of Man* would also have it do (figure 2). The same pair of veins (the "fourth pair") are described as reappearing visibly on the surface of the abdomen after emerging from the liver and spleen, then travelling to the penis and testicles, in the manner of the superficial epigastric veins on the left side of Warrior B (plate 9). It is important, in this context, to remember that the statues did not have interconnective veins from the upper parts of the body to the legs or from front to back in the torso. According to the writer of *Nature of Man*, this would be impossible anyway because the "first pair" of veins are ones which pass invisibly from the back of the head along the spine and then go into the legs, ankles, and feet; they are completely separate from the "fourth pair." The writer's purpose is clear: he wished to show that good health comes from a good Empedoclean mixing of the elements in the body, and so he described the upward-downward, inside-outside, joining-bifurcating anatomy of the veins as proof that nature has arranged for it to happen in the anatomy of the blood vessels themselves. In addition, because he believed that veins begin in the head, he shared the contemporary theory of the brain as the centre of consciousness, as outlined in *The Sacred Disease* (17–20), where transcutaneous breathing and the nutritive notion of respiration are also assumed (7 and 10). The importance of the brain, together with the physiology of respiration through lungs and skin, was vividly dramatized in *On Breaths* (9–10) and further elaborated in a later Hippocratic work of the fourth century, *On the Nature of Bones*. This last work was based on a much older idea derived from Syennesis of Cyprus and Diogenes of Apollonia (fl. 450 B.C.), namely, that the brain is the seat of consciousness. To this idea there was a corollary: the "white" parts of the body, that is, the sinews, nerves, and bone marrow, had their origin in the same place as the blood vessels, namely, in the brain.[40] I would suggest that the effect of parallelism and overlap between sinewy parts, bones, and veins in the hands of the Riace warriors is the visual equivalent of this anatomical idea.

D: SCULPTORS AND PHYSICIANS

The Omphalos Apollo, the funerary stele from Paros, and the Riace warriors thus exhibit some, but not all, of the interpretations of respiration available in the fifth century. This was to be expected. We can remind ourselves again that the sculptors who made them were *not* physicians or philosophers, and they were not students of either physicians or philosophers, as far as is known. They were artists, and as such, they were engaged in using anatomy and physiology to make statues which had expressive and plausible meanings in their physiques, with the intention of satisfying patrons and pleasing audiences at a level of common understanding and response. This is why they were more like effective bone-setters than theoreticians of physique or anatomists. However, even a bone-setter must be aware of the terminology, progression, and movement of the body, and of new discoveries and theories, which professional physicians had described and systematized.

If sculptors were like physicians and philosophers in any way, the closest they ever came was to resemble the speaker who gave the medical speech *On Breaths*. This discourse ("treatise" is too heavy a term for it) is an extremely dramatic, short, and well-organized rhetorical essay, full of striking metaphors and impressive literary devices. The text is unusual in the Hippocratic corpus because of its overtly rhetorical character, but as such, it may be typical of medical *paideia* of the fifth century (see above, p. 20). The speaker's purpose was to distil and synthesize concepts for a general audience already receptive and alert to his ideas. Its effectiveness lay, like that of a statue, in brief but vivid enumeration of examples tending toward, but not rigidly oversteering the audience to, a unified theory of medical knowledge and interpretation. *On Breaths* has been criticized, too narrowly, for its mistakes, absurdities, and illogical propositions, but its tone is persuasive and histrionic rather than dogmatic.[41] The speaker credited his audience with enough intelligence to understand many and various kinds of alternative explanations and interpretations of single phenomena, and like Plutarch in the *Parallel Lives*, he let his listeners make up their own minds about the evidence for his arguments.

A similar procedure and spirit, I believe, operated intellectually among the sculptors of the Omphalos Apollo and the Riace warriors. They were eclectic and undogmatic about respiration in their statues, but they were quite anxious to show it. This is how they went about it practically and intellectually. Using the new precision of theories about respiration that were current, they added physiological interpretations of internal processes within the body to their anatomical rendering. They were fully aware that showing internal physiological processes (using the same signs by which physicians and philosophers recorded them) in itself indicated the presence of an animating force, because the proof of its presence and bodily location had by then become completely absorbed in the interpretation of physiological phenomena. Their awareness of these considerations had consequences on their representation of the body: on the mouth, newly opened; on the ribs, now numerous and visible; on the features below the navel, namely, the thick flank pads and swelling abdomen; and on the shape of the iliac-inguinal line, newly redesigned. In choosing to shape the ilaic-inguinal line as they did, they were not, I believe, merely codifying stylistically what had been a previously not-too-stable anatomical feature of older statues. Instead, they were motivated by a desire to express physiological processes, in this case, respiration. They needed a shape which would clearly distinguish between flank pad and abdomen, and between these two and the legs, and further up, between rib and flank pad, so they invented one that would do the job visually.

The sculptors of the Omphalos Apollo and the Riace warriors also understood that the unity of human physique does not derive from an old or a new style dogmatically applied to all parts of the body. Instead, they recognized that the external signs of internal physiology both separate anatomical parts from each other and also unite them, through their rhythms and visible dynamic processes. Hence, the sculptors began to represent the superficial veins, because veins had become the proof of choice for numerous notions about the pre-Socratic soul – in whatever manifestation of animating force was used at the time – and its location in the body, besides being the evidence for respiration.

It seems to me that the sculptors had this great luck: they did not have to commit themselves too firmly as to where the animating force might be. In this respect, they were better off than the physicians and philosophers, who were required (in fact eager) to do so. In addition, the sculptors were lucky, because ultimately, the Socratic formula – that the soul really is non-material and not specific to any locus or substance in the body – would have defeated their efforts at specific depiction. However, they did commit themselves, in these three statues at least, to the general interpretation of respiration and blood as nutritive function. In the fifth century, this commitment may not have excluded all others in the way Aristotle, writing much later, claimed it did. The choice of respiration and blood as nutritive function had two advantages, visual and physiological: it co-ordinated inhalation with pulsation (shown in the fullness of the veins at the extremities), and it made a correspondence between the open mouth and the redesigned lower abdomen. There was a double bonus too: the external points of flexion in their statues could be marked by superficial veins to express internal physiological processes and to emphasize the unique opposite flexion (elbows and knees) of the human body. Two advantages and a double bonus: it is no wonder that the sculptors were eager to depict the nutritive function of breath and blood. It was efficient to do so because with one feature – namely, the veins – they could effectively convey two levels of physical meaning, both human flexion and respiration. In the Omphalos Apollo and the Riace warriors, the meaning of inhalation is thus to show presence of the animating force, existing a priori in the body's physiology and manifesting itself externally.

I believe that the sculptor of the girl in the Paros stele (plate 3) had the same iconographic impetus: to show the presence of the animating force or soul by depicting its principal *semeion*, namely, the physiological process of respiration. He used the means at his disposal: the drapery of the beltless peplos indicated abdominal breath and corresponded to the redesigned lower abdomen in male figures to show inhalation.

In depicting physiological processes, the sculptors of 480–450 B.C. were perhaps also motivated to respond to an attitude about sculpture which appears in the Hippocratic corpus a few years later. The attitude has all the marks of a popular prejudice or, rather, of a chic vulgar quibble about artistic work that gets picked up from generation to generation and day to day and makes the rounds of stoas, along the streets, and finally (and sadly) is repeated to the sculptor in his workshop. The quibble is this: that artists only knew how to show the outside of bodies, but could not represent the soul inside, and therefore they could not represent the body truly, but only according to its external form (*The Art* 12, comparison of medicine to visual art in a broken passage; cf. *Regimen I* 21, on various crafts). The quibble is clearly of Sophistic origin, because intellectually it depends on the popular *nomos-phusis* dichotomy. This is why Socrates, who was allergic to this kind of pseudo-intellectual rubbish and did not much care for Sophists anyway, was so encouraging to Parrhasios the painter and Kleiton the sculptor about their effectiveness and ability to show manifestations of the soul's character and effects in their figures (see p. oo). Socrates, or perhaps we should say Xenophon (who liked Sophists even less than Socrates did), was scoring off the Sophists by showing that artists could, indeed, reveal the soul.

Artists are better off ignoring Sophistic rubbish, but a quibble can sting if repeated often enough, and it can motivate artists to respond to it through their works. If the statues under consideration here constitute a kind of response to the quibble, we should be as grateful for it as we are to the sculptors themselves.

Three anomalies mentioned at the beginning of this chapter remain to be resolved. Two are anomalies between the Omphalos Apollo and the girl from Paros, and the third concerns the Omphalos Apollo only. The first anomaly is the veins in the male figure and their absence in the girl, and the second is the large head of the girl in relation to the small head of the Omphalos Apollo. The third anomaly is the head-to-body proportions (about 1:7½) of the Omphalos Apollo, somewhat greater, as I have noted, than the proportions (about 1:7) of later standing male figures. As we shall see in two cases, the anomalies are only apparent, and the visual differences between and among the statues can be reconciled by reference to Greek medical thought.

The interpretation of veins has been sufficiently stressed with respect to anatomy and physiology in the Omphalos Apollo and the Riace warriors. Veins had other interpretive possibilities: they were physiognomic indicators and indicators of the typological varieties of human physique according to various categories (sex, age, place of habitation, race, and so on), besides being indicators of certain physical conditions such as overdevelopment, health, and disease.[42] I will have occasion below to speak again of veins, their aspect and interpretation, and so I limit myself here to outlining how physicians used them as indicators of disposition in men and as differentiating between men and women, in order to resolve the anomalies between the Omphalos Apollo and the girl from Paros.

During the fifth century, physiological speculation was the chief means to understanding the location and activity of the body's animating force, and it is for this reason that it became one of the major concerns for Hippocratic physician-writers. At the same time, physicians had at hand another, apparently plausible, and useful interpretive tool, that of the humours (*khumoi*).[43] I have omitted discussing the humoral theory with respect to Greek statues because it was undergoing lively revision and mutation throughout the fifth century, and its form as we think of it today (and as we use its terminology) is quite different from what it was for the Hippocratic physicians, for Aristotle, and for the Peripatetics. In Greek times, the nearest it got to the medieval and Renaissance *Vierschema*, or rigid four-part system, was when it appeared, perhaps around 400 B.C., in *Nature of Man*, primarily chapters 1–8.[44] As we have seen, this treatise is based on Empedocles' theory of the four elements (with Love and Strife) making up the soul; the physician elaborated this into a loose, but somewhat dogmatic, system of blood, phlegm, yellow bile, and black bile, seasonal considerations, moist/dry-hot/cold balances, and so on. In his mild dogmatism, he was not generally followed by many other physicians or philosophers, as he is the first to admit, rather disarmingly (2.1–5). Other Hippocratic writers wavered among primacies of various humours and sometimes added more. Plato certainly did not commit himself, and neither did Aristotle or his followers (cf. *Timaeus* 86d–e; *Physiognomics*, passim). This lack of common agreement did not come about because the physicians and philosophers were unwilling to be dogmatic when necessary; it was because the humoral theory itself resisted dogmatic manipulation in the state it was in at the time.

In part, the imperviousness of the humoral theory was a result of the fact that phlegm and yellow bile seem to have been latecomers, whereas blood and black bile had been in residence longer, and of those two, the condition of black bile, in general emanating from the liver, had been early recognized in association with blood.[45] It is the only clearly named humoral condition in the Hippocratic collection called *Aphorisms* (4.9) – melancholia. The taxonomy of the other humours was a later development and does not even appear with any great precision in *Nature of Man*. Moreover, until the fourth century, when the blood vessels, as Plato and Aristotle decided, came from the heart, the liver could also be one of the sources of blood; in *On Nutriment* (31), the arteries are said to be rooted in the heart (by arteries was meant the interior blood vessels), whereas the superficial veins visible on the body's surface are rooted in the liver. A variation on the idea is found in *The Sacred Disease* (6), where, significantly, the veins of both legs and both feet, together with all the superficial veins on the *right* side of the body and the head, emanate from the liver;

these veins are larger and more numerous than those on the left (which come from the spleen).[46] In general, the right side was the positive side in Greek thought, anatomically stronger and physiologically more active than the left side, and its superiority included the inner organs (cf. Aristotle *Parts of Animals* 671b.28–37).

The references are not numerous, but their currency is confirmed in later references to veins and blood in men and women that may have been based on the early association of liver and blood, the right side, and the superficial veins. Melancholia is a disposition of the soul and a condition of the blood, and an indication of its presence is great prominence of veins, with the corollary that veins, as we have seen, can also contain air and be part of the nutritive function of respiration (*The Sacred Disease* 10).[47]

In a section of *Problems* (sometimes attributed to Aristotle himself) where the melancholic disposition is discussed, the writer collected, listed, and tried to explain some old and common notions about melancholy, ones to which he did not necessarily subscribe himself (953a.10–957a.35). He also seems to have found melancholy very heavy going, as Peripatetics did in all those discussions in which there was an obligation to begin with mythological, literary, and historical figures (Heracles, Ajax, Lysander, Empedocles, and others) who could not be empirically verified. In any discussion of melancholy, of course, citations of great men were indispensable, because melancholy was the chief characteristic of great men, poets, and philosophers. The writer's discomfort with the issue of melancholy was broader, because he quite exceptionally contradicted his master's (or, if Aristotle, his own) statement about its nature: in *Problems*, it is said that melancholy is a mixture of hot and cold, whereas in other passages it is said to be cold only and thereby chilled the blood (*On Sleeping and Waking* 457a.31–4; cf. *Problems* 874b.17–20).

Internal contradictions in an uncomfortable Aristotle or Peripatetic writer notwithstanding, melancholy, being associated with blood, was naturally found in small, dark men whose flesh is hard and dry and whose veins stand out prominently (*Problems* 954a.6–8; cf. *Regimen II* 64.12–14). Women are said to have, paradoxically, more blood than men, even though their bodies are smaller, but the blood is on the inside of the body and is for that reason not manifested in the superficial veins (*History of Animals* 521a.22–31). In early Greek medicine, female anatomy was regarded as phlegmatic, moist, and soft, and the only reference in the Hippocratic corpus to prominence of superficial veins in women is remarkably telling: women who are small, dark, and hard of flesh and who exhibit visible superficial veins are the easiest to impregnate and the most fertile, because obesity and moistness, which are the natural dispositions of females, naturally discourage conception and fertility (*Airs, Waters, Places* 10.34–6 and passim; *Regimen I* 27; *Prorrhetics* 24). In other words, women who were anatomically most like melancholic men were notably fertile. It takes little to deduce the corollary: all melancholic men have unusually high sexual drive and frequent, fecund ejaculations (*Problems* 878b.38–39, 880a.30)!

The notion seems to have been that women as a rule did not have superficial veins (except for especially fertile ones, who were considered to be very unusual). Whether this line of thought precluded women anatomically and physiologically from being melancholic, and thereby reduced their capacity for greatness along the lines of Achilles, Lysander, Empedocles, and company, our sources do not say.[48] What is clear is that the absence of superficial veins on women was a matter of their natural anatomy, and thus it is no anomaly that the girl from Paros and other female figures in Greek sculpture do not have veins: on medical grounds anyway, it would be most unusual for them to have them. Thus, their difference from male figures in this respect is not only a stylistic difference, but a matter of current anatomical interpretation. It was impossible for the girl from Paros to have superficial veins, and she shared this characteristic with her other Greek sisters in art, medicine, and natural philosophy.

Turning to her external proportions, that is, the head-to-body proportions of about 1:5 (plate 3), the Hippocratic writings do not help us much because, since the physicians tended to generalize, they did so almost exclusively about adults and usually about male anatomy as the highest norm of physique from which inferior physiques could be extrapolated. Children's and women's anatomies, as well as their physiologies, were assumed to be inferior. In *Regimen I*, children were characterized as moist and warm, whereas men at the acme of their development were dry and cold, and women in general were moist and cold (33–4). These characteristics of children and women received great elaboration in other contexts, particularly with reference to the explanations of sleeping, its purpose, how it comes, and what it does (*Regimen II* 60). Ultimately, Aristotle developed an etiology of sleep from his sources and investigations which, like the Hippocratic writers, classed sleep as a process similar to digestion, both of which modified the hot/cold-moist/dry balance in the body (*On Sleep and Waking*, passim).[49] It is probably this etiology of sleep which suggested to him that children, in fact, were dwarfs and like dwarfs, had excessively large heads and arms, slept a great deal, were prone to epilepsy, and had inconspicuous veins and bad memory, besides having poorly developed legs (*On Sleep and Waking* 457a.4–10, 22–6; *Progression of Animals* 710b.11–17; [Aristotle] *On Memory and Recollection* 453a.32–b.8). In these passages, the etiology of sleep and digestion was connected to the proportions of dwarfs and children. The connection suggests, as I have said, that Aristotle was using a Hippocratic source such as *Regimen II* to help formulate his idea, and in view of the well-developed association of dispositions which he cites, it may be that his source also contained a suggestion of dwarf physiology in children. If so, it would help us explain the proportions and certain other characteristics of the girl in the stele.

The girl from Paros is unusual in Greek art; she is not depicted like most children in archaic art, who are generally shown as small adults, but she has the face of an adult, quite unlike children in reliefs of the fifth and fourth centuries, where the physiques are generally those of adults, but with faces having fuller cheeks, thicker necks, and snub noses, for reasons which Aristotle explained in great detail (noses: *On Sleep and Waking* 457a.17–19; necks: *Problems* 963b.14–15).[50] The girl cannot be compared to representations of dwarf children or adult dwarfs, who are invariably grotesque in ancient art.[51] I would suggest that the artist of the stele, who, as we have seen, took a great interest in internal physiology, may have extended his interests to include an external proportioning for his figure that reflected a current explanation of pediatric physique, namely, that children were dwarfish, as proved by their physiological processes. Thus the large size of the girl's head, in comparison to smaller heads of other Severe style figures, is only an apparent anomaly. Medically, it corresponded to the dwarfish interpretation of children, and it would not have been considered an anomaly by the artist or by a physician at the time.

Finally, the unusual head-to-body proportion of about $1:7\frac{1}{2}$ in the Omphalos Apollo (and types derived from its original) raises the issue of external proportions, most often called *summetria* in Greek. External proportions in statues, the guarantee of their beauty and formfulness, was a matter of great importance, but emphasis on them by sculptors as a teaching tool, or *paideia*, comes only in the last third of the fifth century at the earliest. Polykleitos was the main promoter of the study of external proportions, and after his floruit, his proportional codes or others like them came to be mentioned by philosophers (Plato *Sophist* 235e–256f; *Philebos* 64e; Xenophon *Memorabilia* 3.10.3). Of course, it needs no repeating that the philosophers held generally negative opinions on the validity of these proportional codes, referring to them as little better than lies or misrepresentations about real beauty, which is itself invisible and anyway irrelevant to human physique. Still, it was Plato and Xenophon who made external proportions in statues (as opposed to human beings) a valid topic of intellectual discussion in philosophy, if rather briefly. Codes of external proportions represented the sculptors' co-optation, from philosophical discourse, of teleological method, that is, of "seeing through" the proportions themselves to divine or universal values and processes. Philosophers, especially Plato, were perhaps jealous of sculptors' abilities to do this, or perhaps philosophers were vexed at the sculptors' co-optation of a bit of philosophical discourse. Whatever the case may have been, Plato was certainly very cross that the teleological method should be borrowed by sculptors in this way, and he made it his business to utter sour remarks on what he regarded as pretentious claims about the codes of external proportions developed by sculptors, even though he did not mention the topic very often.

For sculptors, external proportions were of greater importance than they were for physicians or natural philosophers, either in the fifth century or later. In fact, theories of human proportion are virtually non-existent. No mention of them is made in the place where we would expect to find them, namely, the *Timaeus*, where human anatomy and physiology are analysed teleologically in great and wild detail. External proportions are not discussed at all by Hippocratic physicians. Anything approaching the Polykleitan formulae of modular relationships within a system of proportion is absent from medical literature through Hellenistic times, and it is virtually absent from Peripatetic texts as well; the only thing that the writer of *Problems* says about proportions is that men with large heads are unintelligent, whereas those with small heads are intelligent (*Problems* 955b.4–8). The statement is unelaborated and not rationalized systematically, and although it is presented as definitive, it seems to be too general to be useful in this context. Later, the Peripatetic corollary was that, as proof of their inferior courage, women were cited as having smaller heads than men (*Physiognomics* 809b.4–7). But in the fifth and fourth centuries, at any rate, the head-to-body proportions, or any other system or code of human proportions, seem not to have been under discussion as such by physicians, even as a norm toward which they could generalize; philosophers did not make much use of proportional relationships either.

Instead, and in great contrast to Galen and other, later writers of the Roman period, both Greek physicians and philosophers were greatly interested in the taxonomy and meaning of the internal proportions of the body, most particularly the relationship of parts in the torso.[52] Unfortunately, the discussions do not resolve the stylistic anomaly of the proportions of the Omphalos Apollo *vis-à-vis* the later classical canon, so the small size of his head will have to remain an anomaly for the time being.

However, if we view his proportions in the context of medicine and natural philosophy in the first half of the fifth century, we are in a good position to see why the later classical systems of external proportions, or any other systematic code of bodily relationships, would not yet have been used. A theory of proportions which allowed ideally beautiful figures to be made and a code by which the theory could be successfully applied and manifested in statues are, for sculptors, a theory and code of knowledge and cognition – what is called "knowledge theory," or *Erkenntnistheorie.* Knowledge theory typically folds both ideas and the cognition of ideas into one seamless whole, creating a unified field in which human observation of phenomena merges with divine or universal realities; Polykleitos's ideas on proportions as formulated in the 430s are a good example of such a unified field of observation and a claim to be expressing the reality of an otherwise invisible beauty. Concern with knowledge theory is not much manifested in Greek natural philosophy before Socrates, and it became a major concern only in Plato and philosophers after him. Before that, cognition and knowledge had not been unified in the successful and rigid way that they would be in the late fifth century.

Earlier medical thinkers and natural philosophers – and, I would add, sculptors in the early classical period – were thinking differently, in less unified, more eclectic ways and in ways which emphasized freshness of observation and plausibility (rather than justifiability) of interpretation. Hence the not infrequent allusion, by philosophers, to things such as water-clocks to explain breathing (as Empedocles) or to rotating liquid in bowls to explain primary motion (as Anaxagoras); these homely, familiar, and mechanical illustrations are clues to the variety and diversity of intellectual approach among pre-Socratic philosophers, at a time when unified knowledge theories had not yet created a standard of philosophical discourse. Given this open intellectual situation, sculptors in the early fifth century were similarly eclectic, and while they helped themselves to new ideas and interpretations about the body, they did not let themselves be held down to any specific set of rules. As we have seen in some detail, the location of the animating force in the body and analyses of the physiological proofs of its activity were indispensable to questions of physique in medical literature. Before about 450 B.C., not all of the ideas on these matters had been resolved, but they *had* been thought about, and the sculptors were able to use some of them in their statues. The alternatives of interpretation remained fairly consistent through Aristotle's day; the Pneumatic theorists, as well as Anaxagoras, Empedocles, and many others, had laid out the basic ground quite solidly. What was yet to come in late fifth century were systematic, but intrusive attempts to apply theories of knowledge and cognition to the older medical ideas and practices and, for that matter, in philosophy as well. The intrusion of knowledge theory into medicine was precisely what the writer of *Ancient Medicine* was complaining about, sometime after Socrates had begun to question the prevailing canting formulae about knowledge theory. The correspondence between the cool views on prevailing knowledge theory in *Ancient Medicine* and Socrates' criticisms of the excessive rigidities of the Sophists is not coincidental: knowledge theory was the major intellectual problem of the day.[53]

Ultimately, in medical thinking during the second half of the fifth century and in the fourth century, the whole problem of internal and external co-ordination of parts of the body was revised in the light of systematic knowledge theory as propounded by the Sophists, Socrates, and others. This was also the revisionist procedure of the later Hippocratic movement in general, in which systematization along philosophical models came to be indispensable. Intellectual procedures in medicine became rigorous and dogmatic, even though these procedures did not lead to any more agreement among physicians about the body than the older medicine and philosophy had. What dogmatic procedure did do was to bring eclecticism, experimentation, and undogmatic intellectual behaviour into disrepute. I believe it affected sculptors as well.

Sculptors, prompted by prevailing intellectual ideas, began in the late fifth century to systematize their knowledge of the body and their techniques of physical representation. For this reason, physique in male nudes in the high classical period developed rigidities and dogmatisms associated with individual sculptors such as Polykleitos and Phidias, and these individual, systematic methods of representing physique were in turn taught to and used by their students and associates. In the same way, it was rare for two or more physicians in the Hippocratic corpus to agree, because for each one of them, it had become intellectually necessary to express himself dogmatically. That is why the writer of *Ancient Medicine*, in view of the current fad for contradictory ideas, implied that patients should get a second opinion – from him (21)! Socrates tried to create a unified, sensible knowledge theory and to bring some order to ideas and popular notions, where chaos and lack of agreement were conspicuous. It should not suprise us that sculptors in the high classical period behaved in the same way: they were individually dogmatic, but as different from each other as possible, like Polykleitos and Phidias. And in the same way that it became necessary for physicians to write books in order to uphold their systems of knowledge and cognition, the sculptor Polykleitos felt it neccessary to write a dogmatic book on proportion.[54]

The same intellectual trends led to the sculptors' dogmatic cooptation of what had originally been a creative experiment in the design of human physique: the shape of the iliac-inguinal line in the Omphalos Apollo or in another statue of the years just after the end of the Persian wars. Other elements of Severe style physique were not re-used, but this one was taken up as a common reference point from which the sculptors could then disagree among themselves, just as the philosophers and physicians agreed on a technical definition in order to refute one another as to its interpretation. For these reasons, the Omphalos Apollo – its bronze original or another Severe style work – indeed represented an experiment, one which was continued with brilliant intellectual and visual vitality in the Riace warriors. But soon after, *both* rigidity *and* great variety of physical representation become apparent in sculpture, in the same way physicians and philosophers began to behave with respect to conflicting knowledge theories. The "egotism" of the Hippocratic treatises, already in preparation during the fifth century, had a parallel in the sudden emergence of artists with personal styles, careers, names, pupils, artistic progeny, and political, regional, and intellectual filiations; it is only an accident of later editorial practice that we have lost the names of the physicians who wrote the treatises, but in all other respects they behaved in the same way as did the sculptors. It is, assuredly, this "egotism" which creates differences of opinion and ideas among practitioners of the medical or visual arts: in the differences, of course, lay the beginnings of a clear medical and a clear artistic history.

The Omphalos Apollo thus represents a new form of male standing nude, a type created first as an experiment in design to express new ideas about the body and and the manifestation of its animating forces. Subsequently, parts of it came to be dogmatic codes for sculptors of the high classical period.

CHAPTER FOUR

Motion and Expression

By 450 B.C. the medical profession and the sculptors' craft had been absorbed in matters of physiology for a least a generation. For sculptors, the reasons for this absorption lay in the discoveries about bodily design and their application to statues. These discoveries paralleled, in medicine, the physicians' revision of Pneumatic ideas in the light of Empedocles' vitalism and their new interest in veins and respiration, the interpretation of which had become crucial to questions concerning the soul and its effects. The idea that a still body, at rest or in potential motion, could at the same time literally be animate came to have consequences on standing male nudes of the early and high classical periods which were profound, thorough, and quite a change from what has been called the *frühe Bewegung* – the early, rudimentary movement – of kouroi in the archaic period.[1]

The differences between male nudes of the classical period and the earlier archaic kouroi involve the ideology of health as much as developments in style and technique. There is no question that stylistic and technical developments provided links of similarity among kouroi and between kouroi and classical figures. However, the differences between them should not be minimized, and in medical terms, as well as in terms of the ideology of health, the differences are marked in a variety of ways. Specifically, there are two areas of physique which differentiate them: motion and stance of body (discussed in section A below) and face, with characterization of facial expression (section B). However, issues of physique may also have been involved with issues of the identity of statues, their patronage, and their intended audience, and all three factors are involved with the popular and élite culture of health, so it is with these considerations that I begin.

In the sixth century, the actual identity of kouroi seems to have be a generalized one, the statues not representing anyone – human or divine – in any specific way. Sometimes the bases on which a kouros was placed call it an *agalma* ("gift" or "token," by inference, "statue"). Even when the figures – such as those of Kroisos and Aristodikos – represented individuals, they did so in what seems to be a generalized way. In contrast, early and high classical figures may well be individualized, as in the case of portraits, and the male nude after about 480 B.C. became either a god or a human being, often a mythological or heroic figure or an athlete with various attributes or in a special athletic position. Specification and individualization had not been the intended iconographic norms for kouroi (and certainly not their visual norm), in part because of the conditions of their patronage: they were meant to commemorate individuals or an act of piety, signified in statues privately commissioned by members of a family, social class, or tribe or by a local government, itself constituted of members of aristocratic governing families.[2] Although some of the dedicators' names are recorded, only one kouros, the "Kroisos" from Anavysos, had the circumstances of his commemoration and death recorded on the statue base, thought somewhat vaguely.[3] The emphasis in the archaic period seems to have been on the act and context of death and commemoration – itself a pious *drama* or ritual deed – rather than on the specific identity of the statue itself. That said, at Athens and elsewhere, the findspots of kouroi are significantly specific: they could be set up in or near temple precincts or in cemeteries.[4] The environment itself provided the context of *drama* for the statues, and it further specified the commemoration of a pious or heroic act.

As such, kouroi should be seen as a outgrowth of the lyric exaltation of *arete*, or personal, prideful excellence, which itself was an adaptation, by aristocratically oriented poets for noble patrons, of the epic personality and scheme of values. Pindar's odes in honour of athletes are the most notable examples of the fusion between lyric culture and aristocratic patronage, but he stood at the end of a long tradition going back at least a century, a tradition in poetry paralleled by dedications of kouros monuments. Like statues, poems can be called *agalmata* (*Nemean* 3.13), and the two may well have been linked in the popular mind. Pindar himself acknowledged the link when he said that he was not a maker of statues (*Nemean* 5.1).[5] The primary meaning of this statement is that his poems were to be heard, not looked at, and he is also claiming that his art is higher than the mere craft of making statues. I would suggest a further meaning: that his poems were about specific individuals and identified biographical circumstances, whereas statues as *agalmata* were generalized and had no or little biographical information. Pindar's gathering of hosts of mythological references to bear on a specific athletic victory – which thus becomes an exemplary pattern of action – was a process which was quite unlike the archaic act of setting up a statue, much less making one.

The dedication by private individuals of kouroi and of other types of statues continued to be made through the last years of the Persian Wars, when the Kritios boy was set up on the Athenian Acropolis, itself always the venue of choice for statues commemorating the pious act of an individual patron. When the Athenians returned to their devastated city in 480/479 B.C., they buried the statues. After that, private dedications virtually ceased at Athens, and because Athens was the model of patronage for Greece in general, they ceased elsewhere as well, except at Olympia and certain other athletic sanctuaries, where individual athletes were still being honoured with statues.[6]

In contrast, the sculptors of the generation of about 480–450 B.C. were the first to make figures whose names were derived from their distinctive action or attribute; their identity was important, as well as their action and iconography. There was a burst of popularity for athletic positions and manoeuvres of all kinds, as represented in statuettes; these small-scale representations, by specifying the pose of the figure, indicate affiliations with a specific athletic contest or training.[7] Myron's *Diskobolos* seems to have been the first of such figures on a large scale, and the *Doryphoros* and *Diadoumenos* of Polykleitos, though not in specific athletic poses, are later instances of this kind of identification. Such statues are no longer *agalmata*: they are not generalized tokens and their creation was not a matter of commemorating pious acts by specfic patrons. We do not know if such statues had specific divine or human identities – Achilles, for example, has been suggested as the "name" for the *Doryphoros*, but this must remain suppositious. However, in the case of the *Doryphoros*, the statue's specific identity (if it had one) could be also be absorbed by its ideological content, in which it became an example of an ideal proportioning or system of beauty. As such, the statue came to be known by the title, *Kanon*, of the book Polykleitos wrote about it in the 440s or 430s B.C.[8]

In the case of these three statues, the patronage situation is not clear, in contrast to the archaic kouroi and korai, whose patrons were often named. Furthermore, because the locations of the statues – where they were set up for viewing – are not known (again in contrast to the archaic statues), there are no clues for the intentions of their patrons and by whom they were to be seen is not known. Polykleitos's *Doryphoros* could have been kept, for some time at any rate, in the artist's own possession, to be used as a record or as a teaching model. Where it was exhibited, if at all, is not known.[9] A change in the market for art may have occurred: certain artists might have been able to support themselves with big commissions, such as the ivory and gold statues which both

Polykleitos and Phidias executed, and as a consequence they might have made other statues "on spec" (as Praxiteles later did; Pliny *Natural History* 36.20) or else for themselves and their students. Such statues would have had an identity and an exemplary intent, and they would not have been subject to the earlier neccessity of being set up to memorialize the piety of a patron. In turn, patrons in the later fifth century may have been intellectually prepared to commission, and artists prepared to make, statues in specific athletic poses or with specific human, heroic, or divine identities and to put the act of commemoration in a secondary position rather than in first place, as had been the case with kouroi.

The new willingness to represent specifically identified, but not commemorative, figures who were at the same time exemplary was, in the fifth century, compatible with contemporary intellectual phenomena in natural philosophy and medicine. The Sophists made uncompromising *arete* old-fashioned, since it had been set aside, at Athens at any rate, by the pressure on individuals of the new democratic politics and morality. This view was also compatible with the Sophists' notion that personal, social, and political behaviour could be guided by principles applicable to all human situations, regardless of individual circumstances, personality, or social status.[10] Socrates ultimately became a forceful exponent of this idea, raising it to a systematic level by calibrating individual and social behaviour along the lines of universal principles of motion and order. He seems to have combined cosmology with natural philosophy and ethical principles in a particularly convincing way, but he was doing what others had done before him.

There is no reason to think that sculptors, together with their patrons and audiences, were uninfluenced by contemporary intellectual events. From the sculptors' point of view, there were some practical decisions to be made about how to represent bodies which would make their statues welcome in a new intellectual situation. They turned to the natural philosophers and the physicians, themselves newly allied, to help them with their decisions. We have already seen how respiration and veins were incorporated into statues on the basis of current medical speculation. The sculptors also sought to incorporate some new ideas about motion and the teleology of human physique as well. Their efforts resulted in, among other things, a new bodily stance and a new definition of the face.

A: MOTION AND STANCE

Motion – its nature and origin – were crucial issues in ancient philosophy; they came to be so in cosmology and anatomy as well. The principles of motion had been under investigation since the seventh century, when the Ionian scientist-philosophers had speculated on the causes of earthquakes. By the end of the sixth century and intensifyingly through the fifth, the nature and origin of motion had developed into a sophisticated series of propositions that ultimately provided the basis of Plato's and Aristotle's ideas on the subject. In addition, speculation on motion could be involved, as we have seen, with the principal involuntary movement in the body, respiration. The connection was made because, by the time Anaxagoras of Clazomenae was lecturing and writing at Athens (c. 460–430 B.C.), the notion that physiological movement and cosmological movement derived from a shared cause had become accepted: Anaxagoras taught that mind (nous) was the initiator of motion, and mind was in both human beings and in the universe.[11]

Motion had also come to be a matter of geometric demonstration and mathematical proof by the mid-fifth century, possibly following the great prominence given to such proofs by the Pythagorean philosophers and by Zeno of Elea (fl. 460 B.C.). Zeno and his teacher Parmenides caused a sensation in intellectual circles at Athens when they went there to lecture in the 460s. During this visit, Zeno presented his famous arguments "against motion," devised to challange and discredit Pythagorean notions of time and space. Four (of some thirty) of Zeno's arguments have come down to us. The best known is that of Achilles and the tortoise; with it and others, Zeno challenged the Pythagorean assumption of indivisible *minima* (or atoms) in space and time by "proving" that Achilles could never catch up to a tortoise to whom he had given a lead (Aristotle *Physics* 239b.14). In turn, Anaxagoras, who took up the Eleatic mode of lecturing and became the most prominent philosopher at Athens from about 460 through the 430s, devised a systematic history of motion. His notion was as follows: a primal, cosmos-creating symmetry and a primal, rotatory motion were replaced, but never fully extinguished, by the present asymmetrical, linear, left-right–up-down–front-back movement of the observable world. *Nous*, the initiator of all motion, had evolved in some way from an original symmetry and rotatory state to a linear state when it came into conjunction with matter.[12] In the matter of popular reception of such matters, the habit of giving nicknames may not be unimportant in estimating the import of a thinker or a work of art: Anaxagoras was nicknamed "Nous" after his guiding notion, in much the same way as Polykleitos's statue was nicknamed "Kanon."

These cosmological speculations and the like may seem to have little to do with sculpture. However, they did provide the intellectual basis for the theories of exercise promoted in the Hippocratic treatises called *Regimen II* and *Regimen III,* most clearly in the former. *Regimen II* is intellectually and rhetorically based on a continual vivid comparison between things static and things in motion. The treatise begins with descriptions of the effects of (static) prevailing temperatures on racial character and health, continuing with a consideration of winds (motion) on the same. Exercise represented motion in the body, and the topic of exercise was presented after a discussion of the invariable (static) effects of certain foods in raw or cooked form and of the effects of sleep and baths. Exercises of sight, hearing, voice, and thought were discussed first (61): exercises of sight, for example, are said to warm and dry the soul, those of hearing to make it vibrate, exercises of thought to consume moisture and make the soul and the body thin and dry, and so on. The author-physician then treated the effects of walking, running, jumping, and other forms of bodily motion, with a system of mathematically measurable results as to the effects of these exercises on the moisture, heat, dryness, and coldness of the physique (66). The point here is that, like the natural philosophers, the physician who wrote *Regimen II* was thinking along the lines of relationships expressed in mathematical and proportional terms, for a readership already alert to using or understanding such terms.

Physical attributes and conditions of motion exhibited themselves in geometric terms as well. Empedocles had distinguished between the primal sphere and its symmetrical motion, as opposed to the physically symmetrical, but planar and – in terms of movement – asymmetrical human body.[13] In this context, Aristotle quoted a fifth-century philosopher (Eurytos?) who defined the boundaries of circles and triangles on analogy to skin and bones in human beings and to bronze or stone in a statue (Aristotle *Metaphysics* 1036b.8–9). By mid-century, as we have seen, Anaxagoras was contrasting primal, universal rotation with the present earth-bound linear movement, in order to compare geometric entities (circles, squares). He proved the properties of the two different kinds of motion with practical demonstrations and examples, such as rotating liquid in a cup or explaining the annual inundation of the Nile. He was actually criticized for the homeliness and vividness of his demonstrations, for histrionically vulgarizing his science; this criticism should, if anything, alert us to the popular effectiveness and ease of understanding which he was after (Simplicius *Physics* 164.17). In fact, it seems to have been Anaxagoras who created the standard of discourse about cosmology: that cosmological speculation should have homely, clear, easily understood geometric demonstrations of universal principles, with interesting and plausible analogies drawn from observable phenomena. His lectures at Athens were apparently famous for such analogies.[14]

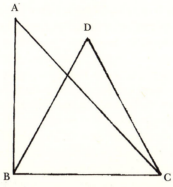

Figure 3. The difference between a right triangle and an isosceles triangle, which Aristotle uses to illustrate the need to bend the leg when walking. AB = BD = length of leg. BC = ground-line. D, the apex of the isosceles triangle, must be lower than A.

Aristotle seems to preserve two of Anaxagoras's proofs, or something not unlike them, in his discussion of human locomotion (figures 3 and 4). Both proofs are presented by Aristotle in contexts and with a brevity which indicate that they were well-known, easy-to-understand commonplaces, and both proofs have the capacity to relate human movement to the geometry of cosmological motion.

1 The first proof concerns the neccessity of bending the leg at the knee to effect walking. A large body, such as that of a man, must have long legs; Aristotle conceived of "normal" proportions as ones in which the legs were as long as the torso, neck, and head. That being the case, he described motion as the difference between a right triangle and an isosceles triangle: a step consists of a transition from the former into the latter and a return to the former, in a geometrical sequence that necessitates bending at the knee and lowering of the apex (in this case, the head) of the triangle (figure 3; *Progression of Animals* 708b.27–709a.24).

Aristotle's discussion is set in a teleological context which has distinct overtones both of the Pythagorean "lists" of good and bad physical properties and of Anaxagoras's idea of asymmetry in nature and motion. He says that "progression," that is, the geometry of animal movement, is made up of six elements in three pairs: upper and lower parts, front and back, right and left (*Progression of Animals* 704b.11–22). Given these elements and a few other particulars, all movement becomes a function of geometrical rules, such as that of bending the knee to effect locomotion. Ultimately, Aristotle will show us why the upper part, the front, and the right side are "better" than the other parts of the body, specifically in terms of human motion, and he will do so because his readers expected it of him, having gotten used to the much older, fifth-century tradition that these parts were indeed superior.

2 The second geometrical proof incorporated a crucial Aristotelian principle: motion is caused by an unmoved mover. All of Aristotle's ideas emanate from this principle, be they cosmological, ethical, or scientific; this needs no recapitulation (*Physics* 258b.4–9). For animal movement, the geometrical proof comes in comparing the movements of the diameter of a circle to that of the radius of the same circle: the centre point of the circle is the unmoved mover for both the diameter and radius, and it is considered, geometrically, to be at rest (figure 4). Thus, the elbow must be considered to be at rest with respect to the movement of the forearm, even though it itself may be in motion with respect to the body, and the body in turn is in motion, and so on (*Movement of Animals* 702b.12–703a.36; for the geometry of internal movement, ibid., 703b.2–704b.2).

The point for Aristotle of the latter proof was to refute the philosophical contention that all things are in movement; in doing so, he aligned himself with Plato, Anaxagoras, and the Pythagoreans in positing a cosmos *and* a human body which have something immovable in them, be it a fulcrum such as the elbow or an unmoved mover such as the soul, which, being unmoved, moves the rest of the body.[15]

Both of these proofs about human motion clearly set aside the physical stance of archaic kouroi in favour of the asymmetrical distribution of weight on one leg (*contrapposto*) characteristic of fifth- and fourth-century standing male nudes. Aristotle's first proof, that of the right and isosceles triangles, also proves the necessity for bending at the knee, something which standing male nudes after the Kritios boy all do and which all earlier statues conspicuously did not. Aristotle also repeated the point that Anaxagoras had made a century earlier: the body may seem to be symmetrical from the outside, but its motion, being timely and earth-bound, cannot be. This last point makes nonsense of the stiff-legged, left-leg-forward stance of kouroi, which would be geometrically impossible in Aristotle's first proof because it would make one leg longer than the other. The archaic stance would also have been impossible according to the standards of functional anatomy described in the Hippocratic treatise *On Joints*, in which even a minute difference in length of leg (due to birth defect or injury) is shown to have consequences on gait, local muscle development, and posture (*On Joints* 52–9). The foot position of kouroi, in which the heel and ball of both feet are flat on the ground, would have been diagnosed in the

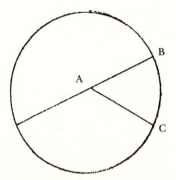

Figure 4. The common-point (A) for both the diameter and the radius of a circle illustrates Aristotle's notion of the unmoved mover in human locomotion.

Hippocratic corpus as the result of an unreduced or improperly
reduced luxation or a poorly set fracture (*On Joints* 60). A mathemati-
cian would have diagnosed the stance of kouroi as a geometrical
impossibility.

That much of the preceeding is merely obvious or in some way com-
monsensical to us or that it would have been obvious in some practical
way to any artist, patron, or viewer in the fifth century is not the point.
By the mid-fifth century, obviousness, common sense, practicality, and
the notions arising from them came under vigorous critical assessment
and evaluation, be it in the domain of the geometry of motion or in the
area of accurate anatomical description using a consistent and developed nomenclature. Probing at the most broad and at the most minute
levels is the intellectual picture at this time, both for physicians and for
natural philsophers. Sculptors, it seems to me, were not so stupid as to
neglect the current intellectual situation.

Aristotle's second proof – that movement originates in something
unmoved – favours classical *contrapposto* in figures at rest, because *contrapposto* is a moment both of rest and of potential movement. In
figures in movement, moments of stillness within movement are
illustrations of the unmoved-mover principle, because stillness is the
fulcrum for motion, either potential or actual. Figures which exhibit
such moments of stillness in their bodily postures are those of the
Severe style and of the early years of the high classical period, that is,
the god from Artemision and the *Diskobolos* of Myron, both presented
in moments of stillness within a narrative of violent movement. These
figures are influenced by a theory of motion involving the idea of an
unmoved mover or its equivalent, and such a theory would have been
compatible, by the second quarter of the fifth century, with both
Pythagorean ideas and those of Anaxagoras.

Anaxagoras's influence on statues, be it direct or indirect, is not verifiable as such, even though he was one of the principal intellectuals and lecturers at Athens in his day. However, a statement which all ancient writers attributed directly to him seems to have been taken up in the Athenian artistic milieu around the same time as he made it; philosophers and sculptors may have moved in the same social circles and may have been prompted to similar conclusions. Anaxagoras, as we have already seen, thought that it was the possession of hands which made man the most intelligent of all beings (Aristotle, *Parts of Animals* 687a.7). The statement was apparently further specified by an observation compatible with his notion of asymmetry in the present universe: hands are the best and cleverest of all bodily parts because nature divided them into fingers of unequal length, and this structure in itself imparted wisdom and understanding to man (Plutarch *On Brotherly Love* 2). The asymmetry of the hand, and its association with the asymmetry of present time and motion in Anaxagoras's view of these things, was one of the traits which he identified as distinctively human in human anatomy.

A striking feature of archaic kouroi is the strangely awkward and unanatomical definition of the back of the hands, knuckles, and first joints of the fingers. In the early sixth century, hands fisted against thighs, such as those of the Sounion kouroi and the Metropolitan kouros (plate 13), have their first knuckles at the back of the palm all aligned parallel to the base of the statue and first joints aligned at about a 45° angle to it. The result was that the first phalange of the index finger was always excessively long, longer than the first phalange of the middle finger. At this period, there were two other alternatives to the design of the hand: hands could exhibit aligned first knuckles and first phalanges all of equal length with a shorter thumb (as in Kleobis and Biton), or knuckles and first phalanges parallel to one another but with a thumb longer than the fisted hand (as in the kouros from Tenea). After about 550 B.C., kouroi with fisted hands almost invariably have aligned first knuckles and first phalanges at a 45° angle, with an excessively long first phalange for the index finger, in the manner of the Sounion kouroi.[16] Curiously, this design of aligned first knuckles and elongated first phalanges of the index fingers occurred in bronze figures with extended fingers as well, namely, in the Piraeus Apollo of about 530 B.C. and in the Piombino Apollo. The latter is a statue which was intended to be in a late archaic or early classical style, but which was made in the Hellenistic or even Roman period. In both these statues, the first phalange of the index finger was longer than the first phalange of the middle finger, as if the fisted hand had merely been extended.[17] In the Piombino Apollo, the index finger is actually longer than the middle finger, and I take this characteristic to be an intentional "mistake" whose purpose was to give an archaic authenticity to the work. The archaic sculptors were thinking of the hand as an amalgam of conventionally patterned parts, and sculptors imitating their works picked up the conventionalizations and used them.

In contrast to the hands of archaic statues, those of figures of the Severe style and later, for example, those of the pediments of the temple of Zeus at Olympia and the Riace warriors (plate 14), all exhibit *unaligned* first knuckles, with the first joint of the index finger slightly shorter than that of the middle finger. This new design emphasized the origins of the fingers' unequal length in the structure of the whole hand, not just of the relative length of the individual fingers. The phalanges of all the fingers are of different lengths, and none follow a neatly aligned profile.

This newly accurate depiction of fingers and joints was a result, no doubt, of the general sharpening up of anatomical and physiological representation after about 480 B.C. However, it may also have been induced by matters under current investigation by natural philosophers. Anaxagoras's preoccupation with the asymmetrical anatomy and function of the hand was an outgrowth of the kind of speculation about physiology and function of other phenomena, such as respiration and veins, which was of great importance in the fifth century. Sculptors, as we might expect, were alert to such speculation, and they used instances of it to bring their works up-to-date.

In the case of the *Doryphoros*, Polykleitos may indeed have been influenced directly by Anaxagoras. They were near contemporaries. In addition, notices of the *Doryphoros* include the fact that its proportions were calculated *down to the very finger joints themselves.*[18] This can perhaps be taken as hyperbole with ironic intent, to ridicule the assiduity of the sculptor in finding formulae for everything in the human body, but such, indeed, was probably his intention. Polykleitos's book about the proportions of his statue, the *Kanon*, was written in the years Anaxagoras was lecturing at Athens and around the time when the philosopher published his single great encyclopedic book, the book in which he considered the anatomy and meaning of the hand and probably other aspects of human proportion and anatomy, besides his ideas of cosmology and motion. Anaxagoras's book was popular enough: it was still available for purchase in Plato's day, though cheaply remaindered in bookstalls at a popular price, earning the philosopher's contempt (*Apology* 26d.1–6).

Returning to the stance of kouroi with respect to that of later figures, Anaxagoras and his intellectual milieu provide a basis for the meaning of *contrapposto* in classical male nudes. As is well known, the asymmetrical stance of figures supporting their weight on one leg seems to have been initiated by sculptors during or just after the Persian Wars: the earliest surviving statue to exhibit the stance is the Kritios boy. In early classical statues, for example, in the Omphalos Apollo, the stance was further developed to accentuate its asymmetry; by the time of the Riace warriors, the stance was fully realized, and while there are variations of detail later on, *contrapposto* in its classical form persisted into Roman times.

Contrapposto is appropriate to still figures. In contrast, it is legitimate to ask what had been represented in the stance of the earlier kouroi. Were they striding forward on their left legs, or were they standing still, left leg forward? It is most frequently assumed that they were shown in a walking position, but this may not have been the case.[19] Their stance may have been intended to show a figure at rest, with the left leg forward for technical reasons – to balance the figure – or for reasons of tradition – to affiliate the figure with the Egyptian origins from which the kouroi are said to have come.

In whatever way we interpret the stance of kouroi, *contrapposto* does indeed differentiate classical figures from earlier ones, on the basis of the legs and the way the weight is carried. Early classical figures in general bear their weight on the right leg like the Kritios boy. The Omphalos Apollo and its types, both Riace warriors, the standing male nudes at Olympia, and most figures in relief of this period are shown standing in *contrapposto* with their weight on the right leg, the left leg slightly bent. In addition, the left foot is slightly in front of the right one. In the second half of the fifth century, in statues of the high classical period such as the *Doryphoros* and the *Diadoumenos* of Polykleitos, the left foot is frequently depicted behind the right one, and after about 440–430 B.C. there is much variation in the foot position of standing male nudes. But in the early classical period, between about 480 and 450 B.C., in statues which were the first to exhibit *contrapposto*, the left foot is shown a little forward of the right.

Medically and in terms of natural philosophy, the stance of the legs, feet, and hips was a developed and teleologically oriented issue in Greek thought. By the 430s B.C. and intensifyingly in Hippocratic treatises toward the end of the century, it is clear that the Pythagorean "lists" of good and bad properties, devised in the late sixth century, had exercised great influence on élite and popular thought. There are numerous instances throughout the Hippocratic writings of physicians demonstrating the superior virtues and strengths of the right side, the upper portion of the body, and its front. In natural philosophy, Anaxagoras and Empedocles were among the first to adopt and to systematize physique along teleological lines. They claimed, for instance, that in human fetuses, the head or the heart developed first (according to where they thought the seat of life might be), and they both agreed that male children are formed of semen from the right testicle, females from the left, and so on (Plutarch *Thoughts of Philosophers* 5.7; Censorinus *On Birthdays* 5.2).

Teleology in physique corresponds closely to iconography in works of art. Such systems assigned both relative and absolute value and meaning to physical processes and anatomical parts, and although at this early period, our knowledge of specific teleological systems is spotty, there is no question that later authors based their systems on earlier, well-developed and influential teleologies.[20]

Aristotle's teleology of motion and physical stance is especially specific. He presented his proofs in a way that indicates that he was relying on popular notions of physical movement, the kind which could be observed in gymnasia and on work sites everywhere. For Aristotle, bodies endowed with an autonomous ability to move were a priori superior to all others, and he cited Anaxagoras as one of his intellectual predecessors who had advanced this claim most successfully. Further to the point, Aristotle asserted that rotatory motion is both more complex than and superior to mere linear motion; this idea was clearly based on Anaxagoras's idea of the primacy of rotation and the secondary emergence of linear motion. Finally, rotation was, for Aristotle, the motion from which time and space are properly calculated. Linear motion was merely a point-to-point device for measuring them (*Physics* 265a.13–266a.9).

From this argument alone, we could not conclude that *contrapposto*, with its suggestion of rotatory motion around the axis of the figure's torso, endowed classical statues with a guarantee that they moved or were about to move in accordance with superior universal motion. As a corollary, we cannot say that the forward movement of kouroi along a line, either actual or potential, would have made them look inferior in the eyes of a fifth-century audience to "modern" figures standing in *contrapposto*. But there is further evidence on the matter, cited by Aristotle in a way that makes such a conclusion unavoidable. On certain matters of human motion, he adduces common knowledge, widely accepted and practically verifiable by anyone. This is his argument in paraphrase:

We all know that it is easier to hop on the left leg than on the right one. In addition, men have a natural tendency to carry heavy loads on their left shoulder, and all men always step off on their left leg when they begin to walk. Furthermore, if we observe tall men, we can see clearly what all bodies naturally do when walking: the back hunches slightly, and the left hip is carried slightly behind the right one. At rest, all men naturally stand with their left foot slightly in front of the right foot (*Progression of Animals* 705b.30–707b.27; cf. *Parts of Animals* 671b.30–7, where the generation of motion from the right side results in internal asymmetry of the organs, e.g., the right kidney is always higher than the left).

For Aristotle, the reason for these phenomena of stance and motion was the innate superiority of the human body, in which upper parts, the right side, and the front are strongly differentiated from their opposites – much more strongly differentiated than the same parts in other animals. In addition, the human body was conceived by Aristotle as being the most in conformity with nature, because the soul, always the initiator of motion in the body, invariably initiated motion from the right side. The consequence was that the first half-step and the weight of burdens were "teleologically" undertaken from the left side, where inevitably there was less potential for movement, in order to leave the right side free to initiate motion and to command the left to follow it (*Progression of Animals* 706b.16).

Intellectually, Aristotle was closely following Anaxagoras's and Hippocratic thinking of the fifth century in his argument about motion, and that not only because of the homeliness and practicality of the examples and illustrations he used – men in gymnasia and on work sites. His emphasis on the asymmetry of external parts and on asymmetrical motion, itself induced by an internal asymmetry inside the body, was fully possible only following Anaxagoras's and the Hippocratic writers' acceptance and assimilation of bodily asymmetry as a structural principle of physique. The asymmetry of the internal organs and blood vessels was a *new* idea when it was first broached by Anaxagoras around 450 B.C., and it was accepted with reluctance. More than a century later, Aristotle himself, in various instances, was still reluctant to dispense entirely with ideal bodily symmetry, and his acceptance of internal anatomical asymmetry was sometimes very grudging.[21]

But for sculptors, the asymmetry of anatomy, and the asymmetrical stance of figures in *contrapposto*, was an exciting new notion. It invested their statues with the authority of two new ideas about physique: that motion, which guaranteed the superiority of animate beings, had an origin asymmetrically located in the body and that the asymmetry of bodily parts (in the hand, in the differences between left and right, upper parts and lower ones, front and back) had some teleological appropriateness, conferring the authority of a new, systematic, and higher conception of nature on their figures.

In sculpture, asymmetry of stance appeared in the Kritios boy about 480 B.C. Asymmetry of physique appeared in medical literature about eighty years later in developed form. In the gap between *contrapposto* in sculpture and the acceptance of asymmetry in medicine stood Anaxagoras's natural philosophy, itself based on explaining asymmetry in time, in motion, and in bodies. For that reason, it is to Anaxagoras, to his immediate intellectual forebears, and to his circle that we can attribute the development and popularization of ideas in natural philosophy which would have given sculptors the aesthetic, anatomical, and teleological field on which to work out the new posture. Anaxagoras's influence on sculpture may have been reinforced by his conviction that the elements of the body, far from being the rather abstract four elements with some other ingredients (as Empedocles had held), were indeed the very things the sculptors were good at representing: skin, hair, bone, blood. Those things were Anaxagoras's "stuffs," or elements of matter; they are the stuff of sculpture too.

Anaxagoras had developed his system of human and cosmological motion by the middle of the fifth century. Physicians took up the ideas and presented them in various Hippocratic treatises later on. They appeared with special succinctness in *On Joints* a little after 400 B.C. In this treatise, the physician-author's intellectual principle was this: all parts of the body have a function (58.83). The principle created a philosophically neat, compact system for interpreting the body, with a teleological reason for reconciling all parts with other ones and for explaining the structures of physique in humans.

For sculptors, it may not have been a simple matter to find a physical stance which combined, in a single pose, all the various components of the many current ideas: rotatory motion as superior to linear motion, the soul or animating force (in whatever interpretation) initiating movement from one side or the other, the authority of what can be observed (such as ease of hopping on the left foot) in relation to the need to represent what was best in accord with nature teleologically. However, as we have seen with the issue of where the impetus of motion was in the body, sculptors were under some obligation to incorporate up-to-date thinking in their works. Their solution, *contrapposto*, undogmatically suggested the varieties and possibilities of current interpretations. *Contrapposto* suggested rotatory motion around the axis of the torso, and it incorporated an asymmetry which was both visually pleasing and also in touch with how philosophers such as Anaxagoras were currently describing the universe and the body. The position at rest, with its specifics of weight distribution and the position of the feet, could be made compatible *both* with current ideas about animating force in the body (which initiates movement from right to left) *and* with the observations about natural stance (as seen at the gymnasium) which bore them out. The external asymmetry of stance in statues also expressed a new notion in current medical knowledge and an exciting new idea: that the internal organs are asymmetrically placed within the torso. Even the hand was remodelled along up-to-date interpretations of its teleological connection with human intelligence.

Earlier, in the sixth century, the tradition of the left leg forward in kouroi may have been maintained because, in Greek natural philosophy at the time, it had been compatible with some early notion of human movement; it may also have been maintained to conform to the notion that the right side was superior. But for later sculptors, those of the early classical period, the anatomical symmetry and the suggestion of linear motion in kouroi would have been the first features to fail the test of modern thinking and of current interpretations about the nature and origin of motion. Medically and in terms of natural philosophy, the anatomy and stance of kouroi must have seemed symmetrical and linear, and therefore earth-bound and not distinctively human.[22]

Contrapposto was developed by early classical sculptors as a bodily design like the devices to depict respiration in the body. The asymmetrical stance and respiration conferred welcome iconographic meaning and the authority of nature on their statues. *Contrapposto* implied *both* universal rotation *and* asymmetry, thus neatly fitting the human body into *both* primal motion *and* present time and motion. It also implied the presence of an animating force in the body as the initiator of motion, either actual or potential, from the right side. The asymmetry of the hand and the asymmetry of the stance were modern representations of new ideas about motion in both the universe and the human body. The writer of *Ancient Medicine* and Anaxagoras must have been pleased.

B: FACES AND EXPRESSIONS

The second area which underwent substantial change in early classical sculpture and which ultimately strongly differentiated classical figures from archaic ones was the structure of the head and the expression of the face. It is the latter which I will treat here.

Classical statues, beginning with such late archaic figures as the Blond Boy, intensifying in the Omphalos Apollo (plate 1), and present also in the Riace warriors (plates 5 and 7), have a curious expression: the eyelids are fleshy and thick and seem to be closing. The expression – a kind of heavy-lidded and sometimes even drowsy look – is always recognizable as the "classical" one, and it is the result of several different facial characteristics, as well as of the shape of the whole head. Heavy-liddedness is not present in all classical heads, nor was it always absent in kouroi, but in male figures it became the norm after the

Kritios boy around 480 B.C. It also became the norm in female figures at about the same time, because korai after the statue dedicated by Euthydikos on the Athenian Acropolis cease to smile and instead have expressions as serious and heavy lidded as their male counterparts. This became the typical expression for statues of both sexes through the fifth century.

In part, the expression is the result of the proportionately lower forehead of all early classical and classical heads relative to the high foreheads of earlier kouroi and korai. It also has to do with the lips. Because Severe style and later heads, both male and female, have lips loosely set in a sad conformation, with distinct downward bowing, a generally pensive expression became the norm, even in statues whose shape of cheeks and chin was different. Modifications occurred with beard, hair, and other specific features, but despite these details, the pensive mouth is virtually universal in statues after about 480 B.C. Even in a statue of famously ambiguous expression, Riace warrior A (plate 5), the baring of the teeth and tongue is curiously combined with a pendulous lower lip and a pensive, downward-bowing upper lip which other classical statues, be they open-mouthed or closed, also have.

Pensive mouths were combined with heavily lidded eyes. It is, of course, the eyes which contributed the most to the classical "drowsy" expression that was stabilized after 480 B.C. In marble statues of males, eyelids were designed with a marked tendency toward fleshiness of both upper and lower lids, a feature which strongly differentiated them from kouroi. Male figures in bronze had the same fleshiness of both eyelids that marble figures had. In addition, bronze statues were equipped with eyelashes set into eyelids which were specially made for the application of metal eyelash inserts. There appear to have been two kinds of eyelash inserts: separate strips of metal sheeting made to fit into grooves cut into the eyelids or wedge-shaped pieces of metal folded over into a cone and clipped at the edges to suggest eyelashes. Eyelash inserts survive in the Delphian charioteer: in that statue, the inserts were of strips of metal sheeting set into grooves. Similar inserts were part of the original eye structure of the Artemision god and the Castelvetrano figure. The Riace warriors had wedge-shaped cones of metal with clipped edges as eyelashes.

Eyelash inserts were invented in the early classical period; they are conspicuously absent in earlier bronze figures, for example, in the Piraeus Apollo. What is remarkable about fifth-century eyelash inserts is that the lower lashes seem to have been of the same thickness, length, and prominence as the upper ones; this is certainly the case in the Delphian charioteer, and the Riace warriors also had eyelashes as abundant above as below. The treatment gives the eyes of classical figures a shadowing which, together with the fleshiness of the eyelids, contributes to their "drowsy" expression.[23]

By the time that a great variety of facial expression had become widespread in Greek sculpture, that is to say, in the third and second centuries, physicians and natural philosophers had also accurately described and interpreted characteristic facial aspects in human beings. These are the sciences of physiognomics, partially preserved in the Peripatetic treatise of the same name (see chapter 1). Drowsiness of expression is, in that treatise, a symptomatic facial characteristic in human beings: it is described as *hypnodesteros to prosopon*, and it is recognized by the following signs, or *semeia*: that the eyes be neither overly "looking about" (staring; *dedorkos*) or anxious (*sunnoun*). The author understood a drowsy expression to be the *semeion* of good spirits, a general cheerfulness, and mental balance: *euthumia* (*Physiognomics* 808a.3–5). The meaning, in the section of the treatise in question, of *thumos* (of which *thumia*, and thus *euthumia*, are derivative compound nouns) is no longer the equivalent of the Homeric "soul of the body" as described in the *Iliad*.[24] By this late date, *psuche* had become the word for soul, whereas *thumos* by then had the value of disposition or soulful disposition, a characterization of general behaviour and external manifestation of the soul. *Euthumia*, in this linguistic context, characterizes a person whose soul's manifestation is generally positive.

Besides the eyes, there were, to be sure, many other facial aspects capable of being interpreted, in addition to the other marks of soulful disposition, of which the *semeia* were to be found all over the face, head, and body. If we were to follow the value scheme of *Physiognomics* very closely, we could say that the drowsy expression of eyes replaced the archaic "smile" of lips of late-sixth-century male and female figures: the pensive mouths of early classical figures no longer needed to smile, as their predecessors had done, because their sleepy expressions were the guarantee and sign that they possessed an innate *euthumia*, the good spirits which may have previously been denoted by smiling mouths.[25]

However, there are difficulties in adopting this interpretation concerning the drowsy look as a sign of *euthumia* in the facial expression of early classical and later figures. The major difficulty lies in the emphasis in *Physiognomics* on soul, a concept which, as we have seen, was not current through much of the fifth century.[26] In part also, the difficulties concern the treatise itself: *Physiognomics* is of a late date (third or second century) with respect to the appearance, about 480–450 B.C., of "drowsy" eyelids and eyelash inserts in statues. Since, as we have seen, treatises in natural philosophy and medicine are heavily dependent on earlier ones, the anachronism might be less serious than would otherwise be supposed, but it would nevertheless require some explanation. In this regard, both sections of *Physiognomics* have an affiliation with an early medical treatise: their closest predecessor, intellectually, in the Hippocratic corpus is *Airs, Waters, Places*, which is genuinely an early work of that collection, possibly datable sometime in the second half of the fifth century.[27] The author of *Airs, Waters, Places* was strongly deterministic and materialistic in his method of describing physique and environment, and in these respects he may have initiated the attitudes later taken up by the authors of *Physiognomics*. At the same time, the intellectual resemblances between the two treatises are not great enough to warrant ascribing well-developed physiognomic "sciences" to the early fifth century, or at least not ones as detailed and as systematic as those developed in the Peripatetic milieu later on.

More serious than the problems of anachronism are the intellectual differences between medical thinking in the fifth century and the later "sciences" of physiognomics. The credibility of physiognomics derives in no small measure from its appeal to interpretations based on static, entirely *visual* observation. Both authors of the treatise point out that one could be fooled by that kind of observation, and both elaborated intellectual protocols to avoid being fooled, but went ahead and used them anyway (*Physiognomics* 806a.19–806b.3 and 809a.2–25). Of course, the authors of *Physiognomics* were operating intellectually at a level well below that of Aristotle and his immediate successors. More to the point, their method (if such it can be called) was certainly not that of the earlier Hippocratic writers, even though the latter were highly different from one another, as we have seen. In all Hippocratic treatises, physicians justly prided themselves on their ability to describe and diagnose on the basis of complex observations of things in motion, flux, and change; intellectually, that was one of the strongest bonds between the physicians and the pre-Socratic natural philosophers, who themselves were concerned with just such phenomena in the natural world. On intellectual grounds, then, it is wise to set aside a purely physiognomic interpretation for classical statues and their expressions, specifically their drowsy look.

Instead, there were other, better kinds of interpretations which are germane to facial expression in the fifth century. As we have found elsewhere, the source for them is Aristotle or writers influenced by him, and as we have also already seen, the nature of the sources is twofold: reports of existing beliefs or notions, and observations interpreted in a teleological way. Aristotle and his immediate followers seem, in both instances, to be relying on earlier sources, closer in date and in intellectual spirit to the pre-Socratic intellectual milieu than the authors of *Physiognomics* were.

Two notions are reported to us about the body, which I present in paraphrase:

The eyes of the head are most like the buttocks and fundament of the body, and the proof of this is that women anoint the eyes to ensure fertility. In addition, the whole face is analogous to the area of the abdomen below the navel and above the genitals; this area is a kind of "nether head" or "nether face" (eyes and buttocks: *Problems* 876a.36–876b.23; "nether face": *On Breath* 485a.19–23 and *History of Animals* 493b.16–25; analogy of eyelids and foreskin: *Parts of Animals* 659b.2–4).

The report of these notions is set in the context of determining the system of analogies among different parts of the body. A system of analogous parts of the physique and a method for determining what the standards of analogy should be are genuinely Hippocratic preoccupations, present in many medical treatises, and they were genuinely pre-Socratic preoccupations as well. The examples are numerous and various. Anaxagoras had discussed an analogy between the mouth and the womb on the basis of his consideration of animal embryology (Aristotle *On Reproduction in Animals* 756b.23–31). The Hippocratic texts abound in notations of correspondences among various parts of the body and in analogies drawn to the crafts, to the state, to machines, and so on, used to explain medical concepts such as the physician's craft, health in general, the physiology of the body, and other topics; the examples cited above are chosen almost at random from Aristotle, but I have provided ones from Hippocratic writings as well (see chapters 1–3). Systems of internal and external analogies are highly consistent both with medical thought and with natural philosophy in the first three quarters of the fifth century B.C.[28]

Systems of analogy among the parts of the body invite reserve of expression in the face; the smiling faces of archaic figures came to be incompatible, I believe, with the new ways of describing correspondences among the various parts of the body. As we have already seen, physiological processes guaranteed the presence of an animating force and denoted its activities: there was no need for a separate facial expression of it. In a situation in which the body, either in actuality or in sculpture, is available for interpretation along lines of analogous structure and function, it is appropriate that the face should, in its sculpted structure, exhibit the regularity and blankness of demeanour which characterize the rest of the body. The sculptors abandoned the archaic facial expression because it was no longer compatible with how their patrons, audience, and they themselves had come to think of the human body, that is, as a field of affinities and analogies among its parts, rather than a structure with expressive parts added to it.

The second notice in Aristotle consists of two teleologically interpreted observations concerning human eyes, presented here in paraphrase:

Human beings are the only animals to have lower eyelashes; a capacity to squint the eyelids is unique to humans (lower eyelashes: *Parts of Animals* 658a.15–16; squinting: *Problems* 896b.5–6 and 960a.1–14).

These observations are plainly culled by Aristotle from a fifth-century source; intellectually, they can only be of that period, for various reasons. They are statements about the body which identify what is unique to human physique. This kind of statement was one which many of the physician-authors in the Hippocratic corpus were given to. In *Regimen I*, for example, human beings are differentiated from animals with respect to their health and constitution, on the basis of the characteristic movement of soul within the body at different stages of development, and in the two sexes; the result was the proposition, by the physician-author of the treatise, of a uniquely human diet for the unique nature of the human physique and physiology.

The physicians were prompted to such statements by natural philosophers in the fifth century, confirmed upon occasion by dramatists. The emphasis on what is unique to human beings found various manifestations. In Aristotle, these particular statements on human eyes are similar to that of Anaxagoras about hands, that the possession of hands confers on human beings the unique intelligence and wisdom which they enjoy. In addition, the observations have the flavour of Pythagorean "lists" of good and bad properties of physique and human nature, and it is the kind of statement which Sophocles turned into verse in the great list of human properties in the midst of the natural environment (the "Essay on Man") which the chorus presented in his *Antigone* (332–72): "language, thought like the wind, and the sense of city-feelings ..." Ultimately, Socrates and Plato will become exponents of precisely this tendency to probe what is unique to human beings in the moral and social sphere, and the idea of uniquely human properties is the premise of Aristotelian thinking as well, notably in such texts as the *Problems*.

It may not be possible to attribute to one specific author the source of Aristotle's statement about human eyelashes and squinting. However, in the context of his texts, it is clear that one of his sources was Anaxagoras's book, either in its original form or in some kind of edited or culled version. There are numerous references to it, as there are in other texts by Aristotle and his followers. Because it is the kind of statement on human uniqueness which Anaxagoras was prone to and because Anaxagoras himself was one of the foremost exponents of this general tendency in the fifth century, it is not impossible that Aristotle had been reading Anaxagoras and had appropriated the observations from him rather than investigating the matter himself.[29]

In this context, the drowsy expression of classical figures takes on a different meaning from that which the author of *Physiognomics* would otherwise have led us to believe. It is not a sleepy look. What the sculptors were trying to convey was not the soulful disposition of *euthumia*, but rather two properties of human eyes which were unique to humans: the ability to squint, or to narrow the eyelids into an intermediate position between fully open and fully closed, and the distinctive possession of eyelashes on the lower lids. Thus, the fleshiness of the eyelids in marble heads provides a broad field for painting plenty of upper and lower eyelashes, and it further conveys the set of eyelids which only humans could possess. The design of the eyes in the few remaining bronze statues of the period shows us what the sculptors in marble wanted to convey: eyelids under tension and eyelashes as abundant below as they were above. Both features guaranteed a lifelike humanness to works of sculpture on the basis of what was thought of as being unique to human physique.

CHAPTER FIVE

Conclusion

The conclusion to a preliminary study can be short because its contents may be of a tentative nature; it is also necessary to suggest lines and areas of further study. Both are presented here very briefly.

Sculptors in the generation after the Persian Wars and in the high classical period were creating works responsive to current intellectual and cultural notions about the body. These notions were themselves based on a combination of tradition and innovation in the ideology of health – of what it means to be in a state of *hygieia* – during the fifth century, among the cultural élites and in popular milieux. As is always the case, health had a changing definition. At the time in question, many different ideas of what health was and what the human body might be for were being formulated, and it is these ideas which later constituted the variety of viewpoints in the Hippocratic corpus. Medical treatises of the late fifth and of the fourth century tell us, in part, what had been formulated earlier; the intellectual alliance between physicians and philosophers, which was forged at this time, allows us to use pre-Socratic natural philosophy as a source for medical and interpretive ideas about human physique.

Among the many questions asked by physicians and natural philosophers in the fifth century, two are of interest to sculptors and to us: What are the manifestations of animating forces in the body? and, What is uniquely human about the human body? There were, to be sure, many answers, almost as many answers as there were physicians and philosophers.[1] However, a reasonable agreement was reached. In answer to the first question, most physicians and philosophers were willing to say that signs or symptoms (*semeia*) of animating forces were externally visible in the body in two ways: in observable physiological processes and in motion. The second question was answered by lists of features which were thought to be unique to humans. Sculptors incorporated some of the areas of agreement into their works.

Respiration (and with it, veins) and motion were among the main manifestations of animating force. The interpretations of what respiration was and whence motion arose might have varied, but all interpreters agreed that both of them signified the presence of one or more animating forces. Showing respiration necessitated redesigning the lower abdomen in standing male nudes and the creation of the iliac-inguinal line, and it necessitated showing veins as well; it so happens that the specific interpretation of veins, as they are shown in statues, supports what was later understood as the nutritive function of respiration and blood. With respect to motion, *contrapposto* was the sculptors' response to the various ideas of motion current in the fifth century. Finally, the design of eyes, eyelashes, and eyelids confirmed what seems to have been one of the items in the lists of uniquely human characteristics.

Sculptors, physicians, and natural philsophers had affinities among themselves in the fifth century, in part because none of them were very far from either the popular notions of anatomy and physiology, which frequently surface in medical literature, or from the milieu of up-to-date interpretations of physical phenomena. The physicians and natural philosophers had the task of translating their ideas into a useful new literary form, that of the prose essay, and the sculptors had the duty to create works embodying the new ideas. The dynamic of change, from the late archaic styles to the look of bodies in the early classical period after about 480, is due to the sculptors' desire to represent the new ideas about the body. These ideas had an iconography because in medicine and natural philsophy they had a teleology: the presence of an animating force and the uniqueness of the human physique could be palpably demonstrated, and both could be related to corresponding phenomena which guided the world and the universe. The change, and the motivation for the change, to what we term a "classic" norm was inspired by new thinking in medicine and natural philsophy, and it is no wonder that the sculptors were anxious to adopt it.

The study of medical literature in Greek and Roman times allows us to understand what was considered to be natural (*phusikos*) at any given period. Together with the indispensable conjunction of natural philosophy, it therefore provides a powerful tool for the investigation of all artistic phenomena, of which a very few have been considered here. The task is facilitated by the character of ancient medicine, which was, as a consequence of its position in society, as much in touch with popular ideologies of health as it was with the newest philosophical interpretations. At no time did it have the esoteric and purely professional isolation from social attitudes and popular behaviour which contemporary medicine can have.

The application of medical history to the history of Greek art can be extended both chronologically and through various media. Our knowledge of medical thought in the archaic period is much more fragmentary than it is for the fifth century. At the same time, the sources for classical medicine used in this study also outline some of the terms of physical and physiological belief, in the sixth century at any rate. Moreover, there is a progressive disengagement of medicine, and thus of the human figure, from the much older norms of the natural embodied in epic poetry. For these reasons, a study of the human form in vase painting, in small bronzes, and in monumental sculpture could very well document the growth of medical ideology in a culture still absorbed in working out its relation to the standards of knowledge enshrined in Homer and Hesiod. Archaic physiques preserved an affiliation with various pasts, but they were made at a time when natural philosophy – new ideas about motion, time, cosmology, and physique – were also being formulated.

For the fifth century, no parallel history of art and medicine is fully complete without a consideration of vase painting and the norms of human physique, motion, and expression that were invented in it. In addition, vase painters illustrated "medical" situations from time to time, but always with the intention of making their illustrations relevant to a culture and to a patronage which might have had intentions and expectations quite different from those of physicians. An example is in a red-figure kylix in Berlin, painted by the Sosias Painter in the early fifth century, which shows Achilles bandaging Patroclus's arm (plate 15). This very famous painting illustrates, through the representation of a "medical" situation, something about Achilles' character: it is a comment on the contrast between his bravery and kindly love for his friend, which are never in doubt, and his ineptness at bandaging. His ineptness is all the more playfully shown in that both the painter and the owner of the vase would have known that Achilles' knowledge of medicine was, in fact, famous since he learned it from his tutor, Chiron the centaur, himself the teacher of Asclepius and Machaon, the Homeric physicians (*Iliad* 11.832). The hero is attempting to apply an over-and-under, X-bound bandage which, if properly applied, could close the wound effectively yet remain loose and comfortable (*In the Surgery* 10). From Patroclus's pained reaction, it seems that Achilles has bound the bandage too tightly. In addition, he has bundled it up in such a way as to get the two bandage ends running in the same direction: the loose bandage end in his left hand cannot be tied onto the unsecured bandage end in his right hand. The whole mess is going to have to come off and be redone properly, preferably by an expert, a real physician! Even though this is a battlefield bandage, intended to do well enough until the soldier can see a medic, the difference of expression between the complacent Achilles and the pained Patroklos adds comic salt to the scene. This piece of "medical" mismanagement on Achilles' part is probably intended to lampoon him and to praise him at the same time: his bravery and kindness are alluded to, yet here we see him failing in a small task of purely manual dexterity.[2] It is no accident – he is simultaneously great and inept.

Another venue for the study of medical content and contexts in Greek art is to be found in the small bronzes of the period, which have been omitted from this investigation. For that reason, this study by no means exhausts the many points at which medical literature and natural philosophy intersect with classical art. Nor does it for large sculpture either. Most notable are the external proportions of the torso with respect to the discovery of the internal asymmetry of the organs. What has also not been considered here is the effect of two new medical techniques on the conception of the human body: palpation (the seizing and handling of internal organs through the skin) and auscultation (listening to the sound, either respiratory or vibratory, of the internal organs). These were ultimately to become descriptive techniques in natural philosophy, as they were to become diagnostic techniques in medicine. The effect of these procedures on the depiction of the torso has yet to be investigated.

Finally, the larger questions of the relationship between works of art and the ideology of health – and the ways in which both change dynamically – are applicable as much to architecture and town planning (where authors in the Hippocratic corpus have some definite ideas about the location and organization of cities) as they are to individual instances of physiognomy displaying character in public situations, such as on Roman imperial portraits and coinage. Another area for medical investigation is in Roman iconography; for example, Hercules in Roman statues is frequently depicted with a corpulent body sometimes covered with veins, whereas Roman Apollos are slim and exhibit a feminine anatomy, and they rarely have veins. In all of these instances, what is needed is both a specific knowledge of the state of medical theory and practice at the time and a way of synthesizing medicine and art through the intellectual devices of current natural philosophy and its correspondences in popular milieux. I have sought to suggest the means of that synthesis in the limited period between about 480 and 450 B.C., but this study can be extended both chronologically and in terms of other media in antiquity.

Is it possible to define with any precision the relation between sculptor and intellectual in the fifth century? In what way were Greek artists related to the world of ideas? The answer to these questions is a various one; there is always the possibility that this is an Occam's razor and that by demanding an over-precise answer, we are distorting the situation and cutting the evidence more finely than it can bear. However, there are at least two areas in which artists and intellectuals can be seen to interact, as well as at least two areas in which artists were indifferent to intellectual promptings or incapable of responding to them or in which physicians were indifferent to artists.

In the area of interactions between artists and intellectuals, it seems clear that the main project of intellectuals in the fifth century, the "inquiry into nature," had consequences on medicine and art, as well as on other aspects of popular and political culture. The framing of the inquiry, stripped of any help from mythological interventions drawn from epic and lyric literature, set up a situation in which a kind of empirical research came into being; in any case, a tradition of criticizing magical, popular, and traditional lore in the explanation of phenomena came to be ingrained among intellectuals. In addition, attempts at establishing distinctions of class and hierarchy within the natural world, and in particular an attempt to identify human anatomy and physiology as special and unique (but still relatable to other natural phenomena), seem to have been made. Physicians evidently kept up with these developments, and they seem to have incorporated some of these ideas into their own notions of health and their description of the body. This may have created a model of behaviour for sculptors in respect of their craft and their view of the human body: a closer attention to details of the human body as contained in lists of special characteristics unique to human beings. Such lists – the Pythagoreans' among them – could well have been generated and discussed in intellectual circles as proper topics for debate. Anaxagoras's "stuffs" – hair, skin, bone, fingernails, and so on, and his explication of them as having discrete and independent natural structures – would have been a good place for sculptors to begin. It is also clear that sculptors were responding to earlier intellectuals and physicians, who had prepared the way for Anaxagoras: the characteristics of the Severe style – its emphasis on the contrast between smooth, soft flesh and harshly metallic hair, its insistence on clear differentiation betweeen skin and bone, and its abrupt, but graceful separation of parts of the body, all more marked than in late archaic sculpture – may be precocious instances among artists of the "inquiry into nature" in Anaxagoras and in the Hippocratic treatises. Although it intensified in the later fifth century and especially during the fourth, the tradition of inquiry was a long one. In the years after the Persian Wars, physicians and philosophers were asking questions about the world and making distinctions about natural forms which sculptors cannot have failed to pick up on; intellectuals and artists were both seeking clear descriptive languages, without mythological or traditional reference, in which to speak.

A second area of artists' responding to intellectuals' and physicians' ideas may be in their addition of iconographical elements to human physique in sculpture – ones which were implicit on or within the body, not props or narratives outside of it or added onto it by the meaning of the place where the statue was located. Sculptors seemed to want to put plenty of natural meaning into the physique of their statues, independent of props.

For this reason, iconography in the sculpted body and teleological tendencies in interpretations of the human body come together in the fifth century, particularly in the answers to two central questions: What is the meaning of motion? and, What does it denote? Ultimately, in the fourth century, motion will denote the presence and action of soul, and autonomous, willed locomotion will come to be the highest physical attribute of human beings. Earlier, in the fifth century, something of the same kind of interpretation of motion in human physique must have occurred to artists: not only did sculptors and their patrons become very intererested in explicit movement (of an athletic type, in many instances), but they also became interested in potential anatomical movement – *contrapposto* – and in physiological processes denoted by motion – respiration, swelling of abdomen, blood, and veins. The basis of classical naturalism was not "clinical," in the sense that sculptors began to see phenomena more accurately; their accuracy was a partial and limited one, prompted by their response to new ideas of animating forces in the body and how such forces were manifested and could be shown in statues. The origins of these ideas lay in the intellectual circles of philosophers and physicians; how artists became aware of these ideas is not certain – we do not know, for example, whether sculptors made a habit of attending public lectures by teachers such as Anaxagoras. But that they became aware of them is clear from their statues. The visible signs (*semeia*) of animating force and of human uniqueness in the natural world – opposite flexion of limbs, lower eyelashes – were there in human beings for intellectuals to explicate, and they were there in statues to guarantee the presence of the things of which they were the *semeia*, or signifiers.

It is precisely at this point, of course, that sculptors became indifferent to further elaboration; it is also the point at which further elaboration became moot. It is not actually possible to show such things as the soul in statues, at least not without specific iconographical props. It can certainly be demonstrated that, later in the fifth century and certainly on Attic and other grave stelai in the fourth century, such things were alluded to. But at the time in question (c. 480–450 B.C.) in the early classical period, explicit depictions beyond those implicit in the bodily *semeia* were not attempted: the signs were enough. That is why the jibe against artists in *The Art* was intended to sting: the jibe – that artists are deficient in their art because they cannot show the soul, but only the externals of the body (unlike physicians, who can presumably describe both) – was obviously developed as a professional joke, or *topos*, among physicians, as part of a defence of their art (*The Art* 12, alluded to in *Regimen I* 21; see above, pp. 59–60). By the time the physicians' jibe against artists was written down in the fourth century, physicians had vastly elaborated their craft intellectually, and they had become proud of their ability at prognosis, at complicated therapies, and at theoretical explication of sickness and of health – they had become professionals, and their status was assured, at least in their own minds. It was these achievements which gave Greek physicians the confidence to make fun of artists; the artists' best efforts at belonging to the intellectual community were relegated, by physicians, to the merely manual or visual activity of observing and recording *semeia*, an activity bereft of the status of theoretical understanding.

It is in the domain of theoretical understanding that we may find the second area of indifference between artists and intellectuals: as craftsmen of physique, sculptors of the first half of the fifth century may, indeed, have had an intellectual status on the level of paramedics – bone-setters, barber-surgeons, and the like – welcome in a tight spot but deferring at all times to the professionals higher up on the intellectual ladder. By the time of the formulation of the Hippocratic oath, this status was – intellectually, socially, and practically – a highly defined one: the oath makes a distinction between giving medical orders (an activity entirely in the privilege of the physician) and actual cutting or other forms of physical manipulation, the latter activity relegated to those who in the Renaissance came to be known as barber-surgeons or surgeon-barbers. The whole thrust of professional medicine in the fifth and fourth centuries was toward such a distinction; the elevation of theoretical knowledge among physicians had, as an inevitable corollary, the relegation of cutting to a manual, less prestigious status, but one which nonetheless required either some theoretical knowledge or else the supervision of someone who had it. It is in this position – that of bone-setters and barber-surgeons – that we can locate sculptors: their knowledge of theory (of whatever kind) might have been either great or slim, but their knowledge of *semeia* was sound. In the early classical period, sculptors may not have needed to know or believe in, or have been conscious of, the intricate reasonings of philosophers and physicians in order to behave, visually, in the best interests of their subjects, the statues themselves; the manipulation of *semeia* in a visual order which corresponded to their patrons' expectations was certainly enough, and the activity of showing *semeia* enough for both Greek artists and us. The sculptors' intentions were their own, but the intellectual context of their medical and philosophical environment in the early classical period prompted their specific recognition of particular antomical and physiological details; these recognitions have been the subject of this study.

Investigation of Greek and Roman phenomena can in part be aimed at a better understanding of ancient literature, either in general or in the way of further specifying the meaning of Greek and Latin words, their contexts, and their affiliations. This study does the latter with respect to a locution in one of the most famous passages of Virgil's *Aeneid.* When Aeneas saw his father, Anchises, in Hades, the ghost enjoined his son to imagine Roman greatness compared to other nations' talents and gifts. Among those for which the Greeks were famous were bronze and marble statuary, rhetoric, and cosmography:[3]

Excudent alii spirantia mollius aera
(credo equidem), vivos ducent de marmore vultus
orabunt causas melius, caelique meatus
describent radio et surgentia sidera dicent.
                                        Aeneid 6.847–50

Others will better sculpt the softly breathing bronze
And will bring lifelike faces from marble (so I believe);
Others will plead better cases, better describe the track of
     heaven with a stylus,
And the stars' risings.

The capacity of Greek sculptors to depict living faces in marble (*vivos de marmore vultus*) is fairly straightforward, and the phrase itself is not difficult to understand, either in Latin or in the context of classical statues in general. But the phrase "will sculpt the softly breathing bronze" (*excudent ... spirantia mollius aera*) is more "poetic" and obscure because the association of soft breathiness with bronze is not immediately obvious. In poetic multivalence, "breath" and "bronze" (in molten form) may be related through the bellows which are used to bring the fire under the crucible to great heat, but the locution is unique in the *Aeneid* and is not found in other Latin literature; it seems to be an original connection of Virgil's. It is clear, from this study, that what Virgil meant to convey was the visual effect of *respiration* in classical bronze statues. This effect had been one which sculptors, prompted by ideas from medicine and natural philosophy during the fifth century, had tried to show. It is no accident that Virgil, who himself was an exponent of the Augustan revival of Greek forms, recognized the prompting and found a noble phrase, *spirantia mollius aera*, with which to report it to us.

Notes

I have followed the convention of placing most citations for ancient literature in the text and those for modern literature in the endnotes. An index locorum follows the bibliography.

The ancient texts have been used in the following editions. For the pre-Socratic philosophers: H. Diels and W. Krantz, *Fragmente der Vorsokratiker*, 7th ed. (Berlin, 1951–54), and G.S. Kirk, J.E. Raven, and M. Schofield, *The Presocratic Philosophers*, 2nd ed. (Cambridge, 1983). For the Hippocratic writers: E. Littré, *Oeuvres complètes d'Hippocrate*, 10 vols. (Paris, 1849–61), and W.H.S. Jones et al., *Hippocrates*, 4 vols. of the Loeb Classical Library (Cambridge and London, 1923), except when there are superior editions of individual works, such as the text of *Nature of Man*, by J. Jouanna. For fourth-century literature: Plato, Aristotle, and others in the Loeb Classical Library editions, except when there are superior modern editions, such as that of Aristotle's *Movement of Animals*, by M.C. Nussbaum. For the texts of Galen, I have used the edition of D.C.G. Kühn, *Claudii Galeni opera omnia* (Leipzig, 1821–26), with their English and Latin titles.

In citing ancient works, I have used the conventional English translations of their titles instead of their Greek or Latin titles, which are equally conventional; the treatise *On Humours*, for example, is not about humours at all.

PREFACE

1 Gill, *Here at the New Yorker*, 116.
2 With her customary perspicacity, Professor Emily Vermeule pointed this fact out to me in her summary of my talk on this topic at the College Art Assocation annual meeting in Boston in February 1987. On the *techne* of physicians, its character for the Hippocratic writers is discussed by Lloyd, *Demystifying Mentalities*, 57–9, and in his "The Definition, Status, and Methods of the Medical Τέχνη in the Fifth and Fourth Centuries"; its extensions in Langholf, *Medical Theories in Hippocrates*; 242–57.

3 See Edelstein, *The Hippocratic Oath,* passim, and Sigerist, *A History of Medicine,* 2:98–9.

4 The question was prompted by an undergraduate student who asked me, after I had pointed out, in the usual way, the Egyptian origins of the left-foot-forward stance of kouroi, what the *Greek* reasons would have been for Greek sculptors to adhere to the Egyptian convention. This question and the "next" question, namely, the meaning of *contrapposto* in the fifth century, are partially answered in chapter 4, section A. of this study. For a consideration of the continuous tradition of naturalism through the fifth century, see most recently Childs, "The Classic as Realism in Greek Art."

5 See McManus, "Scrotal Asymmetry in Man and in Ancient Sculpture," and also Stewart, "Scrotal Asymmetry: An Appendix"; Winckelmann, *History of Ancient Art,* 1:296. I am not aware of the medical source for Winckelmann's conviction that the vision of the left eye was keener than that of the right; Aristotle and Galen assert that both are equally keen. The source may not be a classical one, and I would be obliged to readers if they could alert me to the origin of this belief. I am grateful to professors B. Bergmann and S. Rachootin of Mount Holyoke College for this reference.

CHAPTER ONE

1 Pollitt, *The Ancient View of Greek Art,* 30, 184–5, 258–9; also full text but scattered in Overbeck, *Die antiken Schriftquellen zur Geschichte der bilden-den Kunste bei den Griechen,* 165–6, no. 927, and 322, no. 1701. Pollitt lists the story in two aesthetic categories, *ethos* and *pathos* for the painter Parrhasios and *skema* for the sculptor Kleiton, but omits in the latter what was, for Xenophon at least, Socrates' conclusion to *both* conversations at 3.10.8–9, which includes the phrase *ta tes psuches erga* as the last thing said. The next craftsman whom Socrates visits is Pistias the armourer, and a new topic and dialogue format are introduced, as Xenophon in-tended and as Pollitt correctly shows, that of *eurhythmia* and fitting pro-portion (Pollitt, 169–70). With the painter and sculptor, the correspondence that was made was between the facial and soul-indicating emotions in the paintings and the athletic actions in the sculp-tures; *ta tes psuches erga* sums up both of them – emotion *and* action. See also Preisshofen, "Sokrates im Gespräch mit Parrhasios und Kleiton," and J. Onians, *Art and Thought in the Hellenistic Age,* 55.

All students of Greek art must be grateful to Professor Pollitt for bringing lucid order to Greek aesthetic language, and my remarks are intended as a small supplement, in a different area of concern, to his taxonomy. This study of the relation of medicine to art is an attempt to document "the rôle of Greek medical theorizing as an integral and influential part of Greek culture" (Langholf, *Medical Theories in Hippocrates*, 257). For Greek terminology about the body and its philosophical dimensions, R.B. Onians, *The Origins of European Thought*, remains the most complete account.

2 On the Peripatetic text and the subject itself, surprisingly little has been written. I do not know why the proceedings of the Aristotelian society and the other fora for scholars of Aristotle hardly mention the treatise, and R.B. Onians, *Origins* does not cite it. A good summary of the textual and some of the intellectual issues is to be found in Byl, *Recherches sur les grands traités biologiques d'Aristote*, 264–8. In ancient art history, in the area where its use would be most appropriate, that is, in portraiture, the fundamental monograph on sources, but not on works of art with physiognomical content, is Evans, *Physiognomics in the Ancient World*; see also a very useful summary by Winkes in "Physiognomonia: Probleme der Charakterinterpretation römischer Porträts"; also Yalouris, "Die Anfänge der griechischen Porträtkunst und der Physiognomon Zopyros"; hints in Nodelman, "How to Read a Roman Portrait," and brief consideration in Pollitt, *Art and Experience in Classical Greece*, 178–80, and J. Onians, *Art and Thought in the Hellenistic Age*, 55. Breckenridge, *Likeness: A Conceptual History of Ancient Portraiture*, lists no physiognomic indicators, and his quotation from Juvenal (*fronti nulla fides*) on the title-page is perhaps telling in this regard, because in point of fact the *opposite* was true in ancient portraiture. Equally, physiognomics does not appear in Richter, *The Portraits of the Greeks*, or earlier in Bruns, *Das literarische Porträt der Griechen*. The initiation of a discussion of physiognomics by Evans, Winkes, and Yalouris is promising, especially in view of the difficulty of the text itself (see note 7 below) and the problems of applying the treatise's rigid (and sometimes contradictory) rules to ancient likenesses. In antiquity, physiognomics was a branch of medicine and natural philosophy, as well as a popular means of knowledge. In the latter regard, see Pitrè, *Bibliotheca delle tradizioni popolari siciliani*, vol. 19, *Medicina popolare siciliana*, admirably translated and republished as Pitrè, *Sicilian Folk Medicine*.

3 For the portrait of Pompey, see Poulsen, *Les portraits romains*, 1:39–41, pl. I,1; Schweitzer, *Die Bildniskunst der römischen Republik*; Breckenridge, *Likeness: A Conceptual History of Ancient Portraiture*, 156, fig. 77. For Alexander, see Richter, *The Portraits of the Greeks*, 225–8, figs. 186–91; Bieber, *Alexander the Great in Greek and Roman Art*, 32–4; and Hölscher, *Ideal und Wirklichkeit in den Bildnissen Alexanders der Grossen*; there is an elegant discussion of the subject in Stewart, *Greek Sculpture*, 1:82, 189. As an example of physiognomic language current in Roman times, the wide forehead which Alexander had (Apuleius *Florida* 7) is a distin-

guishing feature of Augustus's portraits and those of the Julio-
Claudians as well; it can be cited with his stiff hair as a *semeion*. I interpret
the dividing and/or opposing frontal locks in Augustan and Julio-
Claudian portraits as a reference to the hair's stiffness without bristle; it
appears in relief on the forehead with greater or lesser emphasis in
various portraits, and it is ultimately derived from the flat cap of stiff, individualized locks on the *Doryphoros*; for Augustus's hair in its various
manifestations, see Brendel, *Ikonographie des Kaisers Augustus*, and Vierneisel
and Zanker, *Die Bildnisse des Augustus*, 50–4. A different effect of deep
relief is achieved in Augustus's hair in his posthumous portraits, for example, the Flavian one discussed in H. von Heintze, "Ein unbekanntes
Augustusbildnis," 143–54, pls. 34, 36, and 37a, b and d. I see a connection
between this portrait in Munich and that of Nero in Worcester on the
basis of their hair; see Breckenridge, *Likeness: A Conceptual History of Ancient
Portraiture*, 197–9, fig. 104; also 226, fig. 118 for Severus Alexander.
For a boy of Augustan connections and date with a little flip of stiff hair
above his right eye, see Vostchinina, *Le portrait romain*, 141, pls. XII–
XIII (no. 8, inv. #A229). The question of Hellenistic precursors to Roman
portraits is broached in Michel, *Alexander als Vorbild für Pompeius, Caesar
und Marcus Antonius*; see also review by Brilliant.

4 For Plutarch's intended audience, see Russell, *Plutarch*, 9–10, and
   C.P. Jones, *Plutarch and Rome*, 49–59.

5 The tradition of speeches praising great men had its origins in Greek lyric
   poetry, Hellenistic rhetoric, and the Roman encomium. Ultimately,
   its most consistent form is the one which it takes in late antiquity, the
   imperial panegyric; for a brilliant analysis of this kind of rhetoric, the
   traditions behind it, its literary procedure, and its social and artistic
   relevance, see MacCormack, *Art and Ceremony in Late Antiquity*.

6 For an account of the dangers of the game of "Animals," see Clark, *Another
   Part of the Wood*, 219–20.

7 The treatise called *Physiognomics* incorporates two texts in the form we
   have it. The first part (805a–808b.11) is more interesting and intellectually more consistent than the second part (808b.12–814b.10), which,
   though more detailed, reads like a laundry list. The editor who juxtaposed the two texts did not bother to stitch them together philologically
   or intellectually, and the dates of both parts are in doubt, though they
   clearly belong in the late Peripatetic milieu, sometime in the third or second century; J. Onians in *Art and Thought in the Hellenistic Age*, 55, implies a direct connection of the treatise with Aristotle and a fourth-century
   date, too early for the treatise but not for the science itself, in my opinion. See also Byl, *Recherches sur les grands traités biologiques d'Aristote*, 264–8.

8 There is a thoughtful brief summary of medical popular culture – which
   as far as I know has had no follow-up, but which deserves one – in

Lanata, *Medicina magica e religione popolare in Grecia fino all'età di Ippocrate*.
For all too brief thoughts on the popular culture of physique, see
Bucci, *Anatomia come arte*, 31–52, and for a remarkable and convincing
analysis of Renaissance and later developments, Hollander, *Seeing
through Clothes*, 18ff.

The historiography of Greek popular culture is quite long because
it can be said to begin with Fustel de Coulanges's *La cité antique*, but Fustel's
method was well in advance of historical method at his time and has
only recently been re-examined. For the historiographical context, that
of Michelet, in which he stood, see E. Wilson, *To the Finland Station*,
7–67, and Strauss, *The City and Man*, 240–1. As Strauss says, Fustel is the
starting-point for many kinds of investigations of historical phenomena, Greek and otherwise, and two notable Hellenists, A. Momigliano and
S.C. Humphreys, have said that what is needed is a new *cité antique*;
see A. Momigliano in Humphreys, *Anthropology and the Greeks*, 177, and
my colleague V. Hunter in a review article, "Classics and Anthropology"; see also Finley, "The Ancient City." At one level, Fustel's method
is the intellectual background for books on Greek and Roman daily
life, many of which are written in the strong French tradition of interest
in *la vie quotidienne*. There are many of these (for example, Robinson,
Everyday Life in Ancient Greece), the most ambitious being recently Ariès
and Duby, *Histoire de la vie privée*, vol. 1. For the classical period, the
best known of this type of book is that by Carcopino, *La vie quotidienne
à Rome*, widely translated and re-edited.

At another scholarly level, the norms of popular notions of space, leisure,
work, butchering, the images of gods who rise out of the earth (*anodoi*),
purchase agreements of houses, marking of allotments, the cost of
temples, and many other things, that is, the social, economic, and cognitive
terms of everyday life, have been the subjects of remarkably effective
studies by and in the intellectual circles surrounding M.I. Finley, P. Vidal-
Naquet, J.-P. Vernant, R. Martin, and A. Momigliano. Their work is
too extensive to be cited here, so I note only one example for its brilliant
demonstration of methodology and how new facts about the popular
culture can be revealed: Svenbro, "A Mégara Hyblaea: le corps géomètre,"
which convincingly interrelates Greek methods of butchering with social intentions in city planning through a study of the concept of portion
or lot/allotment (*moira*) in Greek; my friend Dr M. Visser is preparing
a study of this concept in Greek literary and popular culture. In a general
way, these studies are variations on and departures from structuralism,
though that designation is too narrow to encompass the range and depth
of these scholars' thought; another approach to culture guiding their
work is modelled on economic history, its modern methods, and the new
ways in which economic documents have come to be analysed. The

semiotic behaviour of artistic phenomena in antiquity has not been much
studied except in architecture: Preziozi, *Minoan Architectural Design.*
An impassioned materialist view of religious popular culture is found in
Bonnard, *La civilization grecque.*

   In instances where Greek philosophers and poets preserved fragments
of the popular culture in their writings, modern scholars have much
more to go on, as, for example, Ehrenberg did in his *People of Aristophanes,*
and as Dover did in *Greek Popular Morality in the Time of Plato and
Aristotle.* Remarkable studies which use the interpenetration of literary
sources and archaeological data also exist, as in Scarborough, *Facets
of Hellenic Life,* and Lacey, *The Family in Classical Greece.* A fascinating study,
because so greatly specialized, is in Hands, *Charities and Social Aid in
Greece and Rome.*

9   For issues of terminology and philosophical ideas with regard to beliefs
about the human body, see R.B. Onians, *Origins.* With respect to the
place of the physician and natural philosopher in a society in transition
from an oral culture to a literate one, a brilliant analysis, on which
in part I base my own ideas of Greek art and medical culture and the relationship of Greek artists to the world of ideas, was made by Lonie
in "Literacy and the Development of Hippocratic Medicine." On literacy
in archaic and classical times in general, see Harris, *Ancient Literacy,*
3–115, 324–5; for the situation at Athens, Harvey, "Literacy in the
Athenian Democracy."

10   See note 7 above.

11   On the treatise, see Hall, *Ideas of Life and Matter,* 1:66–71. Longrigg,
"(Hippocrates') *Ancient Medicine* and Its Intellectual Context," and
Festugière, *Hippocrate: L'Ancienne Médecine,* 58, n.69, posit a date of
420–400 B.C. for the treatise, but a later date, based on a difference
of interpretation of the treatise and the prominence of the *hupothesis*
method which it contains, is convincingly argued by Lloyd in "Who
Is Attacked in *On Ancient Medicine?*" in his *Methods and Problems in Greek
Science,* 49–69. For medicine and philosophy in general, the classic
statements are Edelstein, "The Relation of Ancient Philosophy to
Medicine," and Jaeger, *Paideia: the Ideals of Greek Culture,* 3:3–45; more
recently, Mansfeld, "Theoretical and Empirical Attitudes in Early Greek
Scientific Medicine."

12   Lloyd, "Popper versus Kirk: A Controversy in the Interpretation of Early
Greek Science," in his *Methods and Problems in Greek Science,* 100–20.
Still useful are W.H.S. Jones, *Philosophy and Medicine in Ancient Greece,* and
Longrigg, "Philosophy and Medicine: Some Early Interactions." The
interactions among physicians and natural philosophers on the basis of
cognitive theory is the subject of Beare, *Greek Theories of Elementary
Cognition from Alcmaeon to Aristotle.*

13   Jaeger, *Paideia: the Ideals of Greek Culture,* 1:296–331; Heinimann, *Nomos*

und Physis, 110–69. On the personalities and issues involved, see Mieli, "L'epoca dei sofisti e la personalità di Socrate." The passages in Diels and Krantz, *Fragmente der Vorsokratiker*, dealing with the immediate milieu of Sophists which Socrates knew are conveniently collected and translated in Sprague, *The Older Sophists.*

14 The visits of Socrates to various craftsmen, artists, and other kinds of people in different activities, with a view to conversation and learning, are recorded in most notices of him. There is a striking resemblance between his visits and the long list of crafts and professions to which the art of doctoring is, or is not, comparable according to the writer of *Regimen I,* (12–24). The literary resemblance may well indicate the influence of this or a similar medical treatise on Plato's format and dialogue ideas, because *Regimen I* may be datable to about 400 B.C. or a little later; see Longrigg, "Philosophy and Medicine: Some Early Interactions." It is possible, of course, that contemporary accounts of the Socrates' life and ideas influenced the medical treatise.

15 Edelstein, "The Professional Ethics of the Greek Physician"; more extensive treatment of the topic in Koelbing, *Arzt und Patient in der antiken Welt,* 96–119, and his "Le médécin hippocratique au lit du malade", and in Bourgey, "La relation du médecin au malade dans les écrits de l'Ecole de Cos." On how the profession thought of itself, see Diller, "Das Selbtverständnis der griechischen Medizin in der Zeit des Hippocrates."

16 For a general review of the conditions which qualify health, see Sigerist, *Civilization and Disease*; Henschen, *The History of Diseases.* The most famous study of a specific disease with ecological and social implications is the one by "Malaria" Jones: W.H.S. Jones, *Malaria and Greek History.* On medical geography, see Barkhuus, "Medical Surveys from Hippocrates to the World Travellers"; for a specific instance of an historical disease, Demont, "Notes sur le récit de la pestilence athénienne chez Thucydide."

17 Edelstein, "The Dietetics of Antiquity"; Smith, "The Development of Classical Dietetic Theory."

18 I have omitted consideration of the metaphor of health used with respect to the state, either real or utopian, because it is a large and complex issue in all natural and political philosophical writing; however, see the useful article by Vegetti, "Metafora politica e immagine del corpo negli scritti ippocratici," and R.B. Onians, *Origins*, 426–66, esp. 442–5, where the spatial issues linking the polis with various aspects of physique are discussed.

19 For Heraclitus and his influence, see Wheelwright, *Heraclitus*; for Heraclitan affiliations in the Hippocratic treatise, W.H.S. Jones et al., *Hippocrates*, 1:337–8; I have not seen G. Hofer, "Heraklit, Herakliteer und der hippokratisches Corpus" (Ph.D. dissertation, Bonn, 1950).

20 For the praise of athletes in the context of sculpture, see Stewart, *Greek*

Sculpture, 1:53–4, 109–10, and Day, "Rituals in Stone," 16–28, esp. 22, n.45, 26; for athletic poetry, Burn, *The Lyric Age of Greece*, passim.

21 See in general Finley, *The Olympic Games*, passim and bibliography, xii; there is a fascinating documentation to be found in Young, *The Olympic Myth of Greek Amateur Athletics*. For Athens, see Kyle, *Athletics in Ancient Athens*. An important, highly specialized study is found in Serwint, "Greek Athletic Sculpture of the Fifth and Fourth Centuries B.C."

22 Ashmole, *Architect and Sculptor in Classical Greece*, 29–35; Karouzos, *Aristodikos: Studien zur Geschichte der spätarchaisch-attischen Plastik und der Grabstatue*, passim.

23 An example is the fillet of the *Diadoumenos* of Polykleitos; on fillets, see R.B. Onians, *Origins*, 444–50.

24 Richter, *Kouroi*, 49–50, figs. 78–81; Vatin, "Couroi argiens à Delphes"; Vatin, "Monuments votifs de Delphes."

25 Overbeck, *Die antiken Schriftquellen zur Geschichte der bildenden Kunst bei den Griechen*, 73–109, 113–86, 219–62, 274–304, 386–403; Sellers, *The Elder Pliny's Chapters on the History of Art*.

26 On Lysippos and the Thessalian monument, see in general Robertson, *A History of Greek Art*, 1:468–70, 2:704, nn.55–8, pl. 148a.

27 On *aryballoi* in medical use, the funerary stele in Basel of a doctor with his assistant is the best known; see Berger, *Das Basler Arzterelief*; Castiglioni, "Apothecary Jars in Antiquity."

28 An interesting question can be raised here for fuller discussion in another study, namely, in statues such as the *Apoxyomenos*, which show specific moments of athletic activity, are the hot/cold-moist/dry balances shown by sculptors in their depiction of the body? The visible effects of these balances – and the physical manifestations of, for instance, cooling or heating up – are at issue in many Hippocratic treatises. On anointing in general, see R.B. Onians, *Origins*, 210–12.

29 Maddalena, "Eraclito nell'interpretazione di Platone e d'Aristotole"; Weerts, *Plato und der Heraklitismus*, passim.

30 Heinimann, *Nomos und Physis*, 42–169; Ostwald, *Nomos and the Beginning of the Athenian Democracy*, 20–56; MacKinney, "The Concept of Isonomia in Greek Medicine." For the *nomos-physis* dichotomy in medicine, see Lloyd, "Science and Morality in Greco-Roman Antiquity," in his *Methods and Problems in Greek Science*, 361–4. The Greek development of the idea of nature is brilliantly presented in Lloyd, "The Invention of Nature," in *Methods and Problems in Greek Science*, 417–34. The unhealthiness of athletic conditioning is referred to by Aristotle in *Nichomachean Ethics* 1106b.1–5 and 1147b.31–1148a.4 and specifically discussed as a moral and medical topic by Galen in *Exhortation to the Arts* (*Adhortatio ad artes addiscendas*), 9–10, 13 and *Exercise with the Small Ball* (*De parvae pilae exercitio*), passim. For a comprehensive review of the sources on

the concept of the unhealthiness or immorality of athletic conditioning, see Serwint, "Greek Athletic Sculpture from the Fifth and Fourth Centuries B.C.," 24–38.

31 Lanata, *Medicina magica e religione popolare in Grecia fino all'età di Ippocrate*, uses the same method.

32 On the primacy of vision in Greek thought, see Beare, *Greek Theories of Elementary Cognition from Alcmaeon to Aristotle*, 9–92, 231ff.; sources analysed in R.B. Onians, *Origins*, 76–9.

33 F. Heinimann, M. Ostwald, and G.E.R. Lloyd, cited in note 30 above.

34 This particular section of the *Problems* (895b.31–6) seems to me to be Aristotle's rather than a later Peripatetic addition. The passage, a very interesting one, is not cited in either Pollitt, *The Ancient View of Greek Art*, or Overbeck, *Die antiken Schriftquellen zur Geschichte der bildenden Kunst bei den Griechen*. It is also clear that the author is making delicate fun of Plato since the reference to the bed plainly recalls Plato's bed (*cf. Republic* 596a.1ff.)

35 The conclusions by Serwint in "Greek Athletic Sculpture from the Fifth and Fourth Centuries B.C.," 394–7, 463–7, made on the basis of her examination of fifth- and fourth-century statues depicting athletes, seem definitive: statues of athletes exhibit an air of vigour and health only in generalized ways, and clues to athletic training are not specific. Her conclusions are confirmed by those of Thomas in *Athletenstatuetten des spätarchaik und des strengen Stils*. Of course, it can be noted on general grounds that methods of athletic training result in changes to athletes' physiques, and training itself changes with increasing rapidity. Dolly Stokesay, a protagonist in Wilson's *Anglo-Saxon Attitudes*, is first introduced to us as a professional female tennis player in 1918–19, when training, clothes, and equipment were beginning to make women's tennis interesting; ultimately, she wrote a book about tennis. Since then, tennis and women's tennis have changed to an even greater degree, in large part due to developments in training and clothing. I am told that now many athletes who were successful in a given year of the modern Olympics could not even make their national semi-finals in the next Olympic generation because of the rapid change in coaching methods.

36 Most recently the character of Hippocratic writing with respect to its intellectual stance is raised in Lloyd, *Demystifying Mentalities*, 30–4; for *hupothesis* in medicine, see his "Who Is Attacked in *On Ancient Medicine*?" and "Popper Versus Kirk: A Controversy in the Interpretation of Greek Science," in his *Methods and Problems in Greek Science*, 49, 69, 103–4. The complex nature of generalization in Hippocratic writings is summarized by Bourgey, in *Observation et expérience chez les médecins de la Collection hippocratique*, 109–44, 191–275, and it can be conveniently compared with his *Observation et expérience chez Aristote*, 35–68; cf. Edelstein, "The

Relation of Ancient Philosophy to Medicine," 303 and n.7, where I would see a distinction between generalization and idealization. On the audience and intention of the Hippocratic texts, see Jones, "Ancient Documents and Contemporary Life, with Special Reference to the Hippocratic *Corpus*, Celsus and Pliny."

37 On teleology in Plato and Aristotle's natural philosophy, see Theiler, *Zur Geschichte der teleologischen Naturbetrachtung bis auf Aristoteles*, 65–8, 83–94; on Aristotle, Nussbaum, *Aristotle's De Motu Animalium*, 59–106, and a succinct and elegant statement on Aristotle's teleology and its context in previous natural philosophy in Byl, *Recherches sur les grands traités biologiques d'Aristote*, 155–85.

38 Pollitt, *The Ancient View of Greek Art*, 28–52. In distinguishing generalization among physicians from the teleological tendency among philosophers, I do not wish to make the false dichotomy, first made by Winckelmann, about the development of realism versus idealization in ancient art; for comment on this matter, see Hölscher, *Ideal und Wirklichkeit in den Bildnissen Alexanders der Grossen*, 10–23, 36–42. Rather, I am referring specifically to medical and philosophical situations, not to aesthetic situations *per se*, and it is certainly the case that even this dichotomy is too crude to be completely satisfactory. What is at issue are the tendencies of description and categorization in medicine and natural philosophy that may be applicable to similar tendencies in works of art. This question will be included in a study which goes beyond the present preliminary one.

CHAPTER TWO

1 On this topic, see most recently Lloyd, *Demystifying Mentalities*, 39–71 and Lonie, "Literacy and the Development of Hippocratic Medicine." A fascinating instance is recounted in Sow, "Lecture du paragraphe I du traité hippocratique de la *Maladie sacrée* (ou Epilepsie) à la lumière de la médecine traditionelle africaine."

2 Cf. Lanata, *Medicina magica e religione popolare in Grecia fino all'età di Ippocrate*, 29–45.

3 On sneezing, its antiquity and variety of meanings, and the related manifestations of shuddering, throbbing, and itching, see R.B. Onians, *Origins*, 103–5, 138–40, 196–7, 483, 487.

4 Jouanna, *Hippocrate: La Nature de l'homme*; Jouanna dates the text to 420–400 B.C., but this seems too early. For a date in the fourth century, see Smith, *The Hippocratic Tradition*, 201, 219–21, and nn.56–8.

5 On the many devices of naturalism, its special character, and its several components, the most important recent statement is by Hallett in "The Origins of the Classical Style in Sculpture"; see also Childs, "The Classic as Realism in Greek Art."

6 Lloyd, *The Revolutions of Wisdom*, 102–8; on the theme of public decla-
mation on medical themes, see also Smith, *The Hippocratic Tradition*,
177–222, and Lloyd, "The Social Background of Early Greek Philosophy
and Science," in his *Methods and Problems in Greek Science*, 136–7. A statement of the polemical and rhetorical intentions of a specific manuscript
is to be found in Jouanna, *Hippocrate: La Nature de l'homme*, 38–44,
and is the subject of Ducatillon, *Polémiques dans la Collection hippocratique*.

7 On the Cos/Cnidos issue, see Jouanna, *Hippocrate: pour une archéologie de
l'École de Cnide*, and Thivel, *Cnide et Cos?* passim; most recently, and
tending to downplay the existence of "schools," see Lloyd, *Science, Folklore
and Ideology*, 202ff., and especially Langholf, *Medical Theories in
Hippocrates*, 12–36.

8 The topic was broached by Lanata, *Medicina magica e religione popolare in
Grecia fino all'età di Ippocrate*. It is discussed most recently in Lloyd,
Magic, Reason and Experience, 15–49, and taken up, with respect to the sharing of words between ordinary activities in popular culture and in medicine, in his *The Revolutions of Wisdom*, 203–8. Indirectly, R.B. Onians,
Origins, provides the bases in literary references to the connections
between élite and popular cultures about the body.

9 The promptings – intellectual and professional – for committing medical
theory and knowledge to written form are brilliantly discussed by
Lloyd, *Magic, Reason and Experience*, 10–58, with preceding bibliography.
A return to magical explanations about the body in the fourth century
may have prompted physicians, in reaction, to write on the accumulated
knowledge of three or four generations of medical professionals and
on their own experience, in order to offset what they saw as a regression
in the popular consciousness.

10 André, *Traité de physiognomie: Anonyme Latin*, 59–61 (section 2–12), n.3.

11 An interesting later application can be found in Vikan, "Art, Medicine
and Magic in Early Byzantium." I am grateful to Karen Stanworth for
this reference.

12 I base my statement on the measurements given in Richter, *Kouroi*, 90–157;
colossi of quite different sizes include Sounion kouros, 42–4, figs.
33–9; Dipylon head, 46, figs. 50–3; Kleobis and Biton, 59–60, figs. 78–83,
91–2; Kriophoros from Thasos (unfinished), 51, figs. 84–6; an unfinished kouros at a quarry on Naxos, 154, fig. 592. There is another unfinished male draped figure in a Naxian quarry, illustrated in Ashmole,
Architect and Sculptor in Classical Greece, 19–20, fig. 22. I note that any reduction in size of statues makes the task of sculpting proportionately
quicker by the cube of the reduction rather than by its square, since the
amount of surface to be finished is geometrically, rather than mathematically, less. Most recently, Stewart, *Greek Sculpture*, 1:75, and 2:
figs. 42–3, has proposed that the "popular" size of 1.90 to 2.10 m.
(c. 6 ft.) for standing male statues was somewhat in excess of what may

have been the average skeletal height of Greek males in the fourth and fifth centuries, that is, 1.70 m. If such is the case, then the sculptors are working in a size slightly over life-size.

13 On cultural patronage at the time of Pisistratus, see in general Boersma, *Athenian Building Policy from 561/0 to 404/3 B.C.*. The greater abundance of Attic kouroi is noted in Richter, *Kouroi*, 113, for the period after 540 B.C.; before that, there was a lull (cf. 59, 90) in comparison to the period which had begun in 575 B.C., (75).

14 Aristotle points out in this connection that the tyrant of Samos, Polycrates, broke ground for large temples and public works to create jobs for the unemployed poor (who would support him politically) and to impoverish the rich oligarchs by continual demands for subscriptions to the building funds (*Politics* 1313b.9). The cost of Greek temples has been analysed by Martin in "Aspects financiers et sociaux des programmes de construction dans les villes grecques de Grande Grèce et de Sicile," with astonishing and convincing conclusions, on the basis of Burford's study of the building accounts at Epidauros, *The Greek Temple Builders at Epidauros*. His conclusion is that temples were much too expensive to have been built from the normal government receipts of any Greek city and that all such buildings had to have been built from the plunder of war, the subjugation of others' territories, or compulsory contributions/ taxation, or all three in combination. If this is the case, then the motivation for war and the promptings to taxation assume an interesting nuance in the later sixth century and in the fifth. High taxation and/or compulsory contributions prompt increased productivity from sources of wealth – at this time, mainly agricultural, with primary processed goods (flour, tanned leather, etc.) in second place and manufacture in third. Widespread slavery is a help to productivity in all three areas. Is it possible that the growth of productivity-based wealth in the late archaic and classical periods was in part due to temple building? If so, patronage of sculpture must have come into the picture too.

15 On archaic colossi, see Karakatsanis, *Studien zu archaischen Kolossalwerken*; on fifth-century colossi, Richter, *The Sculpture and Sculptors of the Greeks*, 162–71, 187–8; *testimonia* of colossi in Karakatsanis and in Pollitt, *The Art of Greece 1400–31 B.C.*, 64, 66–76, 90. Later, in the fourth century, colossal statues were frequently made.

16 Byl, "La vieillesse dans le Corpus hippocratique."

17 The issues and differences of opinion about naturalism are well set out in Hallett, "The Origins of the Classical Style in Sculpture."

18 The freshest account of the limner's art and the inadequacies of "going over the lines" is still to be found in chapter 16 of Goldsmith's *The Vicar of Wakefield*.

19 See chapter 1, note 35.

20 The scholarship interrelating art and ideas in antiquity is, of course, too vast to be meaningfully cited here, but perhaps the many books and articles by Webster, notably his *Art and Literature in Fourth Century Athens*, are among the most compelling.

21 On the primacy of ideology and its relationship to the "inquiry into nature," see Lloyd, *The Revolutions of Wisdom*, 109–71.

22 Relief of a horse from Athenian Acropolis (inv. no. 1340): Brouskari, *The Acropolis Museum*, 52, 60, fig. 92.

23 For a list of the representation of blood vessels in statues of human bodies in the early classical period, see p. 33 and note 1 for chapter 3.

24 This is a recurrent theme, so to speak, of Lloyd's many articles in his *Methods and Problems in Greek Science*, most especially in his article "Experiment in Early Greek Philosophy and Medicine," 70–99. In general, see Edelstein, "The Distinctive Hellenism of Greek Medicine," and Schumacher, *Antike Medizin*, 177–211. On shared inadequacies of literary forms and intellectual questions in the Hippocratic corpus, see Vernant, "Remarques sur les formes et les limites de la pensée technique chez les Grecs," and Bariéty and Coury, *Histoire de la médicine*, 76–142.

25 The issue is treated in almost all discussions of Hippocratic medicine; with particular succinctness in Edelstein, Review and "Recent Trends in the Interpretation of Ancient Science," 121–31, 401–39, and in the conclusion of Bourgey, *Observation et expérience chez Aristote*, 147–8. See also Vernant, "Remarques sur les formes et les limites de la pensée technique chez les Grecs," 205–25, esp. 216ff.

26 The nature of facts and the status of empirical observations in general is best explained in Lloyd, *Magic, Reason and Experience*, 126–225.

27 Edelstein, *Die Geschichte der Sektion in der Antike*, and Lloyd, "Alcmaeon and the Early History of Dissection," in his *Methods and Problems in Greek Science*, 164–93.

28 On Heraclitus, see note 19 for chapter 1.

29 Byl, *Recherches sur les grands traités biologiques d'Aristote*, 296–303, 356–70.

30 Of course, bibliography on the *Timaeus* is extensive, but see the analysis in Hall, *Ideas of Life and Matter*, 1:83–103, for differences among the many different interpretations of the dialogue and a comparison between it and Hippocratic texts.

31 Conacher, *Aeschylus' Prometheus Bound*, 48–9, 82–97; I am grateful to Professor Vance Watrous for this reference.

32 A complete discussion of soul and its equivalents in pre-Socratic philosophy is of course not possible. Good reviews of the various definitions – not tabulated as such, but clearly marked out in the discussion – can be found in Pigeaud, *La maladie de l'âme*, 31–70, 525–39, and R.B. Onians, *Origins*, 93–122 and passim. For the soul in medicine, see Sigerist, *A History of Medicine*, 2:84–115; for extensions of *isonomia*, Vlastos, "Isonomia."

CHAPTER THREE

1 Heracles from the Hind of Keryneia metope on the Treasury of the
   Athenians at Delphi: Stewart, *Greek Sculpture*, 1:132, 2: fig. 216, with
   preceeding bibliography. East pediment of the temple of Aphaia at Aegina,
   dying warrior ("der linke Sterbende," O.XI), right striding warrior
   ("der rechte Vorkämpfer," O.II), his enemy ("der Gegner des rechten
   Vorkämpfers," O.III), and right running-crouching figure ("der rechte
   Helfer," O.IV): Ohly, *Die Aegineten*, 1:33–59, 102–13, Beilage A,
   pls. 12–13, 19, 22, 24–5, 66–7, 71, 73–6. Artemesion god: Stewart,
   Greek Sculpture, 1:146–7; 2: fig. 287–8, with preceeding bibliography.
   Aristogiton of the Tyrranicides group in the Capitoline museum:
   Ridgway, *Roman Copies of Greek Sculpture*, 60, pl. 11y, and Richter, *The
   Portraits of the Greeks*, 124 (not illustrated). Still in the classical period,
   but already well into the fourth century, the figures from the temple of
   Athena Alea at Tegea exhibit veins in forearms and at the extremities;
   see Stewart, *Skopas of Paros*, 38.
2 The most useful recent statements are those in the essays brought together
   in Lombardi Satriani and Paoletti, *Gli eroi venuti dal mare*, particularly
   those of Arias, "Analisi critica delle statue"; Paribeni, "Lo stile e la
   datazione"; and Bol, "L'atelier dei bronzi." Arias, Paribeni, and Bol
   disagree substantially with each other on matters of date and style. An
   earlier publication, but one still characterized as "unofficial," is to be
   found in Borelli and Pelagatti, *Due bronzi da Riace*, with the first volume
   on technical data and conservation history and the second on the artistic aspects of the statues. See also Busignani, *Gli eroi di Riace*, with useful
   illustrations. To these must be added Fuchs, "Zu den Grossbronzen
   von Riace"; Harrison, "Early Classical Sculpture"; Houser, "The Riace
   Marina Bronze Statues, Classical or Classicizing?"; Ridgway, *Fifth
   Century Styles in Greek Sculpture*, 237–8; and Ridgway, "The Riace Bronzes,"
   where a date in the first century B.C. is advanced; see also Ridgway,
   Roman Copies of Greek Sculpture, 34, nn.20–2, and 37, nn. 1–2, and 40;
   and Ridgway, "The State of Research on Ancient Art," 8, n.8. A very
   brief anatomical description is found in Serwint, "Greek Athletic Sculpture
   from the Fifth and Fourth Centuries B.C.," 372–5, n.118.
       Mattusch, *Greek Bronze Statuary*, 202–12, presents the most complete
   and comparative technical analysis of the Riace warriors, together with
   a shrewd stylistic summary; she concludes with a date about 460–450 for
   both statues. Earlier, Formigli, "La tecnica di costruzione delle statue
   di Riace," 127 and 140, nn.79 and 80, had suggested a Hellenistic date
   for the arms of Warrior B; di Vita, "Due capolavori attici: gli oplito-
   dromi-'eroi' di Riace," 256, suggested a Roman date for the refec-
   tions. The descriptive anatomy of the statues has been undertaken

by Sabbione in "La statua A," "La statua B," and appendix. The important
photogrammetric diagrams were presented by Sena in "Fotogrammetria dei bronzi di Riace," 227–9, pls. XXXV–XLIV. I note that, like
Sabbione, Sena presents the method and the gadgets used to make
the images, without drawing any conclusions whatsoever from them; why
this should have occurred, I do not know.

3 Poulsen, *Der strenge Stil*: the style is lucidly discussed by Ridgway in *The
   Severe Style in Greek Sculpture*, 3–11, with consideration of previous
   studies.

4 On the Omphalos Apollo statue, see Ridgway, *Severe Style*, 61–2, 81, 103,
   134, fig. 96–7, and bibliography on the type, 74; Ridgway, *Roman
   Copies of Greek Sculpture*, 69, n.25, pl. 81. A list of the fragments of this widely
   copied statue (most armless and headless or else fragments of the
   head, and so not relevant to my discussion) can be found in Johannowsky,
   "Una nuova replica della testa dell' 'Apollo dell'Omphalos' da Baia."
   See also Lorenz, *Polyklet*, 1–18, 21ff. For a copy and a brief consideration
   of other replicas, see Vierneisel-Schlörb, *Klassische Skulpturen des 5. und
   4. Jahrhunderts v. Chr*, 7–15 (#2) and pls. For its location at Athens, see
   Schwingenstein, *Die Figurenausstattung des griechischen Theatergebäudes*,
   52 and nn.5–7. While the stylistic grounds on which this statue has sometimes been related to the sculptures of the temple of Aphaea at Aegina
   are slim, on grounds of physical depiction, its blood vessels and those of
   certain Aeginetan statues (see chapter 2, note 32) bring them close
   together: see Johannowsky, 378, nn.4–5. See p. 35–7 for a discussion of
   the same issue with regard to the arms of Riace warrior B.

5 On this stele, see Ridgway, *Severe Style*, 48, fig. 66, with preceeding bibliography, 48, nn.4 and 55, Tölle-Kastenbein, *Frühklassische Peplosfiguren:
   Originale*, 89–90 (#11f), n.168; Woysch-Méautis, *La représentation des
   animaux et des êtres fabuleux sur les monuments funéraires grecs*, 110 (#68),
   pl. 13; and most recently Buitron-Oliver, *The Greek Miracle*, 140–1, cat.
   no. 28. Tölle-Kastenhein, in contrast to most opinions including mine,
   dates this statue to the late fifth century. There is a stele from Nea
   Kallikrateia in the Thessalonika Archaeological Museum (inv. #6876)
   which is related to the Metropolitan stele and which, in my opinion,
   is similarly attributable to the Severe style; it also shows a young girl in
   profile, with a bird in her left hand. With her right hand, she is holding
   her beltless peplos closed, to prevent it from opening like that of the girl
   in the Metropolitan stele. To emphasize the absence of the belt, the
   apoptygma is also raised in front, and the girl's belly swells against the fall
   of the peplos in a marked way, to emphasize, with less delicacy but
   greater explicitness than in the Metropolitan stele, the inflation of the
   abdomen during intake of breath. The stele is published in Kostoglou-
   Despoine, *Problemata tes Parianes Plastikes tou 5ou Aiona p. Ch*, 89–114,

pls. 30–2, which I have not been able to obtain, and in Woysch-
Méautis, 110–11 (#68a), pl. 13. With respect to the bird, it is possible
that it represents a soul-bird (*ba*-bird; cf. Vermeule, *Aspects of Death
in Early Greek Art and Poetry*). However, this interpretation, while plausible
for late fifth- and fourth-century grave *stelai*, is quite uncertain for earlier works such as the Parian stele, so I follow Woysch-Méautis in her cau-
tious iconographical assessments.

6 Ridgway, *Severe Style*, 11, n.7; the issue of proportions is cited as being one
of the "tangible traits" of the statues, but Professor Ridgway does not
wish to include their "ethos and grandeur" in her discussion of the Severe
style. However, as Pollitt has convincingly shown, such things as "ethos"
and "grandeur" went with the territory in Greek art, were reducible to
meaningful words, and were capable of specific application (*The
Ancient View of Greek Art*, passim).

7 Richter, *Kouroi*, 148–9, figs. 564–9; most recently Hurwit, "The Kritios
Boy."

8 Richter, *Kouroi*, 26, 32–3, 49–50, figs. 9–11, 78–81.

9 Ridgway, *Severe Style*, 45–6, and bibliography, 55; Lullies and Hirmer, *Greek
Sculpture*, 31, 75–6, fig. 133.

10 Richter, *Kouroi*; Piraeus Apollo: 136, figs. 478–80; Aristodikos: 139,
figs. 489, 492–3; Kritios boy: 149, figs. 564–9.

11 Ashmole, Franz, and Yalouris, *Olympia, The Sculptures of the Temple of Zeus*;
Oinomaos (east pediment P): pls. 15, 18; Lapith youth (west pediment Q): pls. 87, 90; Centaur (west pediment N): pls. 98–9.

12 On corporeal definition in medicine, see Roselli, "Problemi relativi ai
trattati chirurgici *De Fracturis* e *De Articulis*."

13 On the peplos and its draping, see Richter, *Sculpture and Sculptors of the
Greeks*, 57–61, and on this relief, Tölle-Kastenbein, *Frühklassische
Peplosfiguren: Originale*, 89.

14 On the stele, see note 5 above.

15 Studies on Pneumatism are extensive. For our purposes, the following
capsulize the situation best: Jaeger, "Das Pneuma im Lykeion";
Maddalena, "L'aria di Anasimene come sintesi"; Wiersma, "Die aristo-
telische Lehre vom Pneuma"; Solmsen, "The Vital Heat, the Inborn
Pneuma, and the Aether"; Kirk, Raven, and Schofield, *The Presocratic
Philosophers*, 146, 158–62; Kahn, "Religion and Philosophy in Em-
pedocles' Doctrine of the Soul"; Hall, *Ideas of Life and Matter*, 1:30–53;
Furley and Wilkie, *Galen on Respiration and the Arteries*, 3–14. For the
relation between Pneumatic theory and proofs of existence, see Verbeke,
"Doctrine du Pneuma et entéléchisme chez Aristote."

16 Pigeaud, *La maladie de l'âme*, passim, but esp. 141–88; Sorabji, "Body and
Soul in Aristotle"; Furley, "Self-Movers."

17 For other beltless peplophoroi, see Ridgway, *Severe Style*, 47–8, 55, fig. 67

(Giustiniani stele [Berlin]); but especially Tölle-Kastenbein, *Frühklassische Peplosfiguren: Originale*, 86–7 (#11b, Giustiniani stele), pl. 53a, 88–9 (#11e, stele from Liatani on Boeotia [New York]), pl. 54b.

18   Richter, *Kouroi*; as a groove in the Melian kouros: 96–7, fig. 274; as a roll in a kouros in Florence: 83–4, fig. 239; as a shadow between planes in the Anavysos kouros: 118–19, fig. 395.

19   Cf. Guralnick, "Profiles of Kouroi." The graphs have no indicator for the profile of the abdomen, but ill. 9 indicates a decrease in the depth of the buttocks in Aristodikos (406–7).

20   "Let's count your ribs" is the ploy my daughter's pediatrician used when he wished her to inhale deeply and hold her breath so he could auscultate her chest.

21   Furley and Wilkie, *Galen on Respiration and the Arteries*, 11–12.

22   For the rhetorical messages of the discourse, see Ducatillon, "Le traité des vents et la question hippocratique," with bibliography; however, her early date is convincingly brought down to 400 B.C. or later by Lichtenthaeler in *Le traité des vents est typiquement pseudo-hippocratique*, 21–2.

23   Many parents try to train their children to breathe "normally" through their nostrils only; they do so in line with Empedocles' view on the matter.

24   Cf. Ioannidi, "Les notions de partie du corps et d'organe"; for the co-ordinating effects of linguistic developments, see the interesting article by Irigoin, "La formation du vocabulaire de l'anatomie en grec." This is in part the subject of R.B. Onians, *Origins*.

25   For a review of the entire ancient literature, see Allbutt, *Greek Medicine in Rome*, chap. 13, and Harris, *The Heart and the Vascular System in Ancient Greek Medicine*, passim. For the Hippocratic material, Duminil, "La description des vaisseaux dans les chapitres 11–19 du traité de la *Nature des os*," but especially her *Le sang, les vaisseaux, le coeur dans la Collection hippocratique*, 15–61.

26   On Pythagoras of Rhegium, see Stewart, *Greek Sculpture*, 1:138–9, 254–5; on veins, Ridgway, *Severe Style*, 22–3 and n.18.

27   See note 25 above.

28   Brommer, *The Sculptures of the Parthenon*, 108, slab VII, figures 52 (marshal) and 54 (maiden). Closer in date to the girl from Paros, the female figures in the Ludovisi throne do not exhibit veins in their forearms, even the bending figures who are helping Aphrodite out of the water: see Stewart, *Greek Sculpture*, 1:149, 344; 2: figs. 306–8.

29   Lloyd, "Alcmaeon and the Early History of Dissection," in his *Methods and Problems in Greek Science*, 179–80; Furley and Wilkie, *Galen on Respiration and the Arteries*, 7–9; Duminil, *Le sang, les vaisseaux, le coeur dans la Collection hippocratique*, 153–234.

30 Hardie, "Aristotle's Treatment of the Relation between Body and Soul";
Ackrill, "Aristotle's Definition of Psuche." Relevant to this issue is the
question asked by I.M. Lonie, namely, "Does the oldest venous system begin
the veins in the head?" to which his answer is negative; see his *Hippocratic Treatises "On Generation," "On the Nature of the Child," "Disease IV,"*
87–97. However, whatever its date, the treatise *Nature of Man* is specific
regarding the origins of the veins. For a general treatment of the location
of the soul, R.B. Onians, *Origins*, 93–122.

31 Richter was the first to make this point, and she was quite right in noting
the "correctness" of the prone and supine attitudes of arms in the extremities of male nudes in the sixth century (*Kouroi*, passim). My point
is that the later Severe style sculptors felt themselves less bound by
these conventions, and they did not hesitate to deviate from mechanical
"correctness" as they saw fit.

32 The Zeus or Poseidon from Cape Artemision has strongly marked joins
of the cephalic and cubital veins in the same position, with, as I see
it, some forward twisting of the elbows to make the joins visible. See p. oo
and note 1 above.

33 Roussel, "La notion de traction dans le *Corpus* hippocratique." On the
potency of knees, see R.B. Onians, *Origins*, 174–80.

34 Cf. Edelstein's view of the physician as craftsman whose creativity and
selectiveness are analogous to those of sculptors ("The Hippocratic
Physician").

35 Kirk, Raven, and Schofield, *The Presocratic Philosophers*, 383.

36 For text and commentary on *Nature of Man*, see Jouanna, *Hippocrate: La
Nature de l'homme*.

37 For Empedocles, a good compact analysis is in Schumacher, *Antike Medizin*,
115–23. See also Hall, *Ideas of Life and Matter*, 45–51, 71–4, for Empedocles and *Nature of Man*. For the treatise *On Breaths*, see Ducatillon,
"Le traité des vents et la question hippocratique," and Lichtenthaeler,
Le traité des vents est typiquement pseudo-hippocratique; see also note 41 below.

38 On the water-clock analogy, see Furley and Wilkie, *Galen on Respiration
and the Arteries*, 4, with bibliography.

39 Duminil, *Le sang, les vaisseaux, le coeur dans la Collection hippocratique*, 74–9,
pl. III.

40 For transcutaneous respiration, see note 37 above. For the anatomy of
the brain, sinews, nerves, and bone marrow, the fundamental article
is Solmsen, "Greek Philosophy and the Discovery of the Nerves," translated
as "Griechische Philosophie und die Entdeckung der Nerven." See
also Clarke and O'Malley, *The Human Brain and Spinal Cord*, 2–10, 140–2.

41 Allbutt, *Greek Medicine in Rome*, 243; Allbutt's criticisms are unjust and ab-
surdly positivistic. See also Ducatillon and Lichtenthaeler (see note 7
above).

42 These are listed in Abel, "Die Lehre vom Blutkreislauf im Corpus Hippocraticum."

43 The origins of the humoral theory are discussed by Bratescù in "Eléments archaïques dans la médecine hippocratique" and "Les éléments vitaux dans la pensée médico-biologique orientale et dans la Collection hippocratique"; among pre-Socratic thinkers, discussion in Lonie, *The Hippocratic Treatises "On Generation," "On the Nature of the Child," "Disease IV,"* 54–62.

44 On the history of the humoral theory, see Schöner, *Das Vierschema in der antiken Humoralpathologie,* 15–76; for a succinct statement, Majno, *The Healing Hand,* 178–80. The classic article on melancholy, blood, and black bile is that of Muri, "Melancholie und schwarze Galle"; see also Flashar, *Melancholie und Melancholiker in den medizinishchen Theorien der Antike,* 21–49, and Jones, *Malaria and Greek History,* 98–101. For the early references to bile, see R.B. Onians, *Origins,* 84–9.

45 Duminil, *Le sang, les vaisseaux, le coeur dans la Collection hippocratique,* 83–5, pl. V.

46 Ibid., 205–71.

47 Flashar, *Melancholie und Melancholiker in den medizinischen Theorie der Antike,* 11–20.

48 For a review of some of the elements of Greek gynecological anatomy in general terms, see Hanson, "The Medical Writers' Woman." It is typical of the way iconography in human culture can come full circle that the image of the single female should ultimately become the emblem of melancholy; this would have made Greek physicians laugh. See Klibansky, Panofsky, and Saxl, *Saturn and Melancholy,* 287ff., 374ff.

49 The relation between Aristotle's Hippocratic sources and his own ideas on the etiology of sleep is outlined in Wiesner, "The Unity of the *De Somno* and the Physiological Explanation of Sleep in Aristotle"; for the relation of sleep to dwarfism and childhood, see Marelli, "Place de la *Collection hippocratique* dans les théories biologiques sur le sommeil."

50 For instance, the peplophoroi girls in the Kleomenes stele (Athens) and the Philostrate stele (St Petersburg) and the naked boy in the stele of Mnesagora and Nikochares (Athens), all with full cheeks and necks and snub noses; see Diepolder, *Die attischer Grabreliefs des 5. und 4. Jahrhunderts v. Chr.,* 10–19, pls. 2:1, 5, and 13:2. The persistent awkwardness of children as depicted in works of Greek art will ultimately need some explaining in terms of the view taken, at various times, of their anatomy, physiology, soul, and health in Greek natural philosophy and medicine and in ancient art in general.

51 Born, "Monsters in Art."

52 The emphasis on internal relationships, as well as the absence of much discussion of external proportions in medical literature, is noted in

Ioannidi, "Les notions de partie du corps et d'organe." Of course, codes of proportions and their theoretical basis in statues has become a challange for scholars, both to crack the code and to interpret the theories. This comes in part because Greek and Latin writers of the Roman period, especially Galen, developed a real interest in these topics. In the gigantic literature on the issue of external proportions in the fifth century, a definitive statement is that in a brilliant work of scholarship by Gregory Leftwich, which meticulously documents the history of Polykleitan proportions with respect to their intellectual filiations in later Greek and Roman times: "Ancient Conceptions of the Body and the Canon of Polykleitos." The most significant contribution in this work is the study of Galen's relatively frequent citation of statues and his familiarity with Polykleitos's *Kanon*, which he may have known in epitomized form. There is, of course, no doubt about Galen's literacy and intellectual abilities. However, Leftwich proposes an equally high literate and intellectual status for Polykleitos's book and statue and posits the influence of a physician and writer, Alcmaeon of Croton, on them. He may well be right, even though the literacy and intellectual status of sculptors before the later fifth century is not, as I show in this study, either as clear or as high as Leftwich proposes for Polykleitos. It may well be that the relationship between sculptors and physicians before Polykleitos's floruit (the subject of this study) facilitated that sculptor's entrée to the company of intellectuals as Leftwich understands it. Scholars anxiously awaiting the publication of Leftwich's material can refer to Tobin, "The Canon of Polykleitos," which points out how the modular system was developed from fine, rather than gross, relationships among parts of the body, a conclusion also confirmed by von Steuben, *Der Kanon des Polyklet*. However, for all these studies, especially Leftwich's, the issue of how reliable – if at all – the Roman copies of the Greek statue are and whether they can properly be used to reconstruct the canonical rules is raised by Stewart in "The Canon of Polykleitos" and the same author's lucid discussion in *Greek Sculpture*, 1:160–2.

53 *Erkenntnistheorie* in Greek philosophy cannot be conveniently capsulized here. In general, see Rivier, "Sur le rationalisme des premiers philosophes grecs," and Guthrie, *A History of Greek Philosophy*, 2:67–70, 97, 228–43, 319, 438–64; a bibliographical listing on the issue appears in Totok, *Handbuch der Geschichte der Philosophie*, 1:77 ff. and passim.

54 See Leftwich's dissertation, cited in note 52 above.

CHAPTER FOUR

1 Kleemann, *Frühe Bewegung*; this study of archaic kouroi is accompanied

by a new and accurate measuring of their proportions and sizes which will ultimately create new standards for the study of them.

2 On the non-specfic identity of kouroi and their aristocratic orientation, see the article "Apollo" in *Lexicon Iconographicum Mythologiae Classicae*, 2:183ff.; Zinzerling, "Zum Bedeutungsgehalt des archaïschen Kuros"; Karouzos, *Aristodikos*, passim; Hurwit, *The Art and Culture of Early Greece, 1100–480 B.C.*, 197–202; and most recently Stewart, *Greek Sculpture*, 1:109–10. There are thorough studies of specific monuments or groups of sculpture in Stewart, "When Is a Kouros Not an Apollo?"; d'Onofrio, "*Korai* e *kouroi* funerari attici"; Day, "Rituals in Stone." I am grateful to a reader for the Canadian Federation for the Humanities for challenging an earlier version of this discussion and suggesting other ways of approaching it.

3 Richter, *Kouroi*, 118, figs. 395–8, 400–1. The base and statue may not go together; see Immerwahr, *Attic Scripts*, 55, no. 287.

4 The findspots are listed in Richter, *Kouroi*; see also Boardman, *Greek Sculpture: The Archaic Period*, 63–4. A sensitive evaluation of the environment of certain of these statues, which could have profited from a consideration of the literary sources, can be found in Osborne, "Death Revisited; Death Revised."

5 On poems and statues as *agalmata* in Pindar, see most recently Fowler, "The Centaur's Smile."

6 For testimonia of statues through the fifth century, see Pollitt, *The Art of Greece 1400–31 B.C.*, 22, 24, 32, 56–8, 91, 93; also Serwint, "Greek Athletic Sculpture from the Fifth and Fourth Centuries B.C.," 63–8, for a tabulation of statues at Olympia.

7 Statuettes of this period showing athletes are documented and discussed in Thomas, *Athletenstatuetten des spätarchaik und des strengen Stils*, passim.

8 For the possible specific identities of these statues, discussion in Stewart, *Greek Sculpture*, 1:149, 160–2.

9 The more famous a work of art, the less is known about its original location, with few exceptions for the fifth century at any rate; it has even been mooted that the *Doryphoros* stood outside the sculptor's house in Argos: see Ridgway, *Roman Copies of Greek Sculpture*, 66, n.2.

10 Much has been written on Sophistical ethics; see the useful summary in Barnes, *The Presocratic Philosophers*, 466–71, 508–35.

11 Schofield, *An Essay on Anaxagoras*, 36–52, which includes Aristotle's notice of the notion; see also R.B. Onians, *Origins*, 82–3.

12 For Zeno and Parmenides, see Booth, "Were Zeno's Arguments a Reply to Attacks upon Parmenides?" and "Were Zeno's Arguments Directed against the Pythagoreans?" For Anaxagoras, see note 11 above and notes 14 and 29 below.

13 O'Brien, *Empedocles' Cosmic Cycle*, 4–54.

14 Gershenson and Greenberg, *Anaxagoras and the Birth of Physics*; Schofield, *An Essay on Anaxagoras*, 25–33, which stresses Anaxagoras's attachment to the Ionian tradition of cosmological narrative and to the lecturing process.

15 It goes without saying that theories of motion are the nails of ancient scientific thought. The topic was the subject of Cornford's inaugural address at Cambridge: *The Laws of Motion in Ancient Thought*. Most recently the entire subject and its doxography have been revised and reinterpreted by D. O'Brien in *Theories of Weight in the Ancient World*; see esp. vol. 1, *Democritus: Weight and Size*.

16 Richter, *Kouroi*, 43–4, fig. 34.

17 See Richter, *Kouroi*, 152, fig. 478, for the Piraeus Apollo; 181, 144–5, figs. 537–9, for the Piombino Apollo. I would argue that the Hellenistic or Roman sculptor of the Piombino Apollo was concerned enough with the kinds of statues and styles he was imitating to include this anatomical peculiarity; the intentional awkwardness of the phalanges of the index fingers would have given authenticity to the statue's physique, in the same way that the quite inauthentic, but archaic-looking, arrangement of the hair was calculated, in this and other statues, to lend authenticity to the work; see a parallel in the hair of an archaizing dancer (National Archaological Museum, Naples, inv. #5604) from the Villa of the Papyri at Herculaneum, illustrated in Pandermalis, "Sul programma della decorazione scultorea," figs. 22–3, 31.

18 Raven, "Polyclitus and Pythagoreanism," 147–52, esp. 151; see also chapter 3, note 50.

19 Hurwit, *The Art and Culture of Early Greece, 1100–480 B.C.*, 196.

20 Theiler, *Zur Geschichte der teleologischen Naturbetrachtung bis auf Aristoteles*, passim. For a discussion of systematic antitheses as applied to works of art, see most recently Stewart, *Greek Sculpture*, 1:160–2.

21 On issues of right, left, and symmetry, see Lloyd, *Methods and Problems in Greek Science*, 27–48. On the general question of symmetry in ancient thought, see von Dechend, "Il concetto di simmetria nelle culture arcaiche"; for the issue of symmetry in Aristotle's anatomy, Duminil, *Le sang, les vaisseaux, le coeur dans la Collection hippocratique*, 123–4, 305ff. Note that in this discussion, I am using the term "symmetry" in its English sense, as the opposite of *asymmetry*, rather than in the Greek sense of *summetria*, which, for works of art, meant proportional relationships.

22 I am avoiding the issue of Egyptian origins for the stance and/or proportions for kouroi; it is not germane to this discussion. The scholar who has most vigorously advanced the claim of Egyptian origins, on the basis of selective proportional studies, is Guralnick, in a series of articles, the most important of which is her "Proportions of *Kouroi*." Her

conclusions may be right, but are, in my opinion, of little actual relevance to what the kouroi had become by the later sixth century. Moreover, it can be noted in another context that the influence of Egyptian medicine on Greek medicine (in the same period that kouroi were invented) was slight; see Saunders, *The Transition from Ancient Egyptian to Greek Medicine.*

23 On the techniques in casting the eyes, eyelids, and eyelashes which differentiate archaic and fifth-century statues and on the eyes and eyelashes of fifth-century bronzes, in general see Robertson, *A History of Greek Art*, 1:182, 187–97; 2: figs. 53b–62d. However, while the Delphian charioteer and Riace warrior A have upper and lower eyelashes, later statues of the late fifth and fourth centuries and those of Hellenistic and Roman times most commonly have upper eyelashes only, at least in bronze; see the technical description of *Augenmontage* and the collections of eyelash inserts published in Bol, *Grossplastik aus Bronze in Olympia*, 93–8, fig. 11, and 135–6 (cat. #425–9), pls. 51–3. A further analysis in Mattusch, *Greek Bronze Statuary*, 183–5, 214.

24 Pigeaud, *La maladie de l'âme*, 443–77; Snell, *The Discovery of the Mind*, 11ff.; Dodds, *The Greeks and the Irrational*, 1–16.

25 On considerations of facial expression in Greek art, see Kenner, *Weinen und Lachen in der griechischen Kunst*. What we interpret as a smile and call the "archaic smile" in the expression of the late archaic kouroi and korai may not have been a smile as we understand it. On some of the varieties of its meaning, see Fowler, "The Centaur's Smile."

26 The fluid use of the concept of *psuche* in *Physiognomics* is an example of the situation that, if the soul had not come about in its Socratic form, something like it would have had to have been invented: it is a concept which simplifies and co-ordinates many different phenomena at both the intellectual and the popular level.

27 Jones et al., *Hippocrates*, 1:120; for a consideration of the date of the early works in the Hippocratic corpus, see Jaeger, *Paideia*, 3:33–6, 299, n.87; and more recently, Ducatillon, *Polémiques dans la Collection hippocratique*, 341.

28 Lloyd, *Polarity and Analogy*, 304–60, and further discussion in his "The Development of Aristotle's Theory of the Classification of Animals," in *Methods and Problems in Greek Science*, 1–26.

29 On the doxographical issues of Anaxagoras *vis-à-vis* later writers, see Gershenson and Greenberg, *Anaxagoras and the Birth of Physics*, 329–78, and Cherniss, *Aristotle's Criticism of Presocratic Philosophy*, 119–20 and passim. For an interesting possible relevance of Anaxagoras's ideas *vis-à-vis* the iconography of the Parthenon frieze, see Stewart, *Greek Sculpture*, 1:159.

CHAPTER FIVE

1 Lloyd, *Magic, Reason and Experience*, 126–225.
2 See Majno, *The Healing Hand*, 148, 542–3, for comment on the bandaging.
  For the further mistake concerning Patroclus's wound, see Daremberg,
  La Médecine dans Homère, 82; on the vase: Griefenhagen, *Corpus Vasorum
  Antiquorum: Deutschland*, 2:7, pls. 49–50; Beazley, *Attic Red-Figure Vase-
  Painters*, 21–2; Burn, *Beazley Addenda*, 1620. I have avoided interpreting
  Achilles in this fifth-century vase as a melancholic, as he appears later
  in *Problems* 953a.10–957a.35, even though general lack of dexterity is a
  prime characteristic of melancholics. Melancholy was not fully developed as a physical and physiological notion when this vase was painted,
  and it was not yet in use as a physiognomic indicator. On the bandage
  itself, a reader for the Canadian Federation for the Humanities perceptively
  suggested its character as a first-aid, field-of-battle procedure rather
  than a regulation bandage.
3 I am grateful to a reader for the Canadian Federation for the Humanities
  for suggesting corrections to my translation; *radio* I take to mean the
  stylus used by geometers to draw proofs.

Bibliography

Abel, K. "Die Lehre vom Blutkreislauf im Corpus Hippocraticum." In *Antike Medizin*, edited by H. Flashar, 121–63. Darmstadt: Darmstadt Wissenschaftliche Buchges, 1971.

Ackrill J. "Aristotle's Definition of Psuche." *Proceedings of the Aristotelian Society* 73 (1972–73): 119–34.

Agnazzi, E., ed. *La Simmetria*. Seminari interdisciplinari di Venezia, no. 3. Bologna: Il Mulino, 1973.

Allbutt, T.C. *Greek Medicine in Rome: The Fitzpatrick Lectures on the History of Medicine Delivered at the Royal College of Physicians of London in 1909–10, with Other Historical Essays*. London: Macmillan, 1921.

André, J., ed. *Traité de physiognomie: Anonyme Latin*. Paris: Les Belles Lettres, 1981.

Arias, P.E. "Analisi critica delle statue [The Critical Analysis of the Statues]." In *Gli eroi venuti dal mare* [*Heroes from the Sea*], edited by L.M. Lombardi Satriani and M. Paoletti, 30–64. Rome: Gangemi, 1986.

Ariès, P., and G. Duby, eds. *Histoire de la vie privée*. Vol. 1, *De l'Empire romain à l'an mil*. Paris: Seuil, 1985.

Ashmole, B. *Architect and Sculptor in Classical Greece*. New York: New York University Press, 1972.

– A. Franz, and N. Yalouris. *Olympia: The Sculptures of the Temple of Zeus*. London: Phaidon, 1967.

Bariéty, M., and C. Coury. *Histoire de la médecine*. Paris: Fayard, 1963.

Barkhuus, A. "Medical Surveys from Hippocrates to the World Travellers." *Ciba Symposia* 6, no. 10 (1945): 1986–7.

Barnes, J. *The Presocratic Philosophers*. Rev. ed. London: Routledge and Kegan Paul, 1982.

Beare, J.I. *Greek Theories of Elementary Cognition from Alcmaeon to Aristotle*. Oxford: Clarendon Press, 1906; reprint, Dubuque, Iowa: University Microfilms, 1966.

Beazley, J.D. *Attic Red-Figure Vase-Painters*. 2d ed. Oxford: Clarendon Press, 1963.

Berger, E. *Das Basler Arztrelief: Studien zum griechischen Grabund Votivrelief um 500 vor Chr. und zur vorhippokratischen Medizin*. Basel: Archäologischer Verlag, 1970.

Bieber, M.B. *Alexander the Great in Greek and Roman Art*. Chicago: Argonaut, 1964.

Boardman, J. *Greek Sculpture: The Archaic Period: A Handbook*. London: Thames and Hudson, 1978.

– *Greek Sculpture: The Classical Period: A Handbook*. London: Thames and Hudson, 1985.

Boersma, J.S. *Athenian Building Policy from 561/0 to 404/3 B.C.* Gröningen: Wolters-Noordhoff Publishing, 1970.

Bol, P.C. "L'atelier dei bronzi [The Workshop of the Bronzes]." In *Gli eroi venuti dal mare [Heroes from the Sea]*, edited by L.M. Lombardi Satriani and M. Paoletti, 77–96. Rome: Gangemi, 1986.

– *Grossplastik aus Bronze in Olympia. Olympische Forschungen*, vol. 9. Berlin: W. de Gruyter, 1978.

Bonfante, L., and H. von Heintze, eds. *In Memoriam Otto J. Brendel: Essays in Archaeology and the Humanities*. Mainz-am-Rhein: P. von Zabern, 1976.

Bonnard, A. *La civilisation grecque: de l'Iliade au Parthénon*. Lausanne: Payot, 1954.

Booth, N.B. "Were Zeno's Arguments a Reply to Attacks upon Parmenides?" *Phronesis* 2 (1957): 1–9.

– "Were Zeno's Arguments Directed against the Pythagoreans?" *Phronesis* 2 (1957): 90–103.

Borelli, L.V., and P. Pelagatti, eds. *Due bronzi da Riace: rinvenimento, restauro, analisi ed ipotesi d'interpretazione*. 2 vols. Rome: Istituto poligrafico e zecca dello Stato, 1984.

Born, W. "Monsters in Art." *Ciba Symposia* 9, nos. 5–6 (1947): 684–7.

Bourgey, L. *Observation et expérience chez Aristote*. Paris: J. Vrin, 1955.

– *Observation et expérience chez les médecins de la Collection hippocratique*. Paris: J. Vrin, 1953.

– "La relation du médecin au malade dans les écrits de l'Ecole de Cos." *Colloque Strasbourg* (1972): 209–27.

Bratescù, G. "Éléments archaïques dans la médecine hippocratique." *Colloque Strasbourg* (1972): 41–50.

– "Les éléments vitaux dans la pensée médico-biologique orientale et dans la Collection hippocratique." *Colloque Paris* (1978): 65–72.

Breckenridge, J.D. *Likeness: A Conceptual History of Ancient Portraiture*. Evanston: Northwestern University Press, 1968.

Brendel, O.J. *Ikonographie des Kaisers Augustus*. Nurnberg, 1931.

Brilliant, R. Review of *Alexander als Vorbild für Pompeius, Caesar und Marcus Antonius*, by D. Michel. *American Journal of Archaeology* 74 (1970): 217–8.

Brommer, F. *The Sculptures of the Parthenon: Metopes, Frieze, Pediments, Cult-Statue.* Translated by M. Whittal. London: Thames and Hudson, 1979.

Brouskari, M.S. *The Acropolis Museum: A Descriptive Catalogue.* Translated by J. Binder. Athens, 1974.

Bruns, I. *Das literarische Porträt der Griechen im fünften und vierten Jahrhundert vor Christi Geburt.* Berlin, 1896.

Bucci, M. *Anatomia come arte.* Florence: Il Fiorino, 1969.

Buitron-Oliver, D., ed. *The Greek Miracle: Classical Sculpture from the Dawn of Democracy: The Fifth Century B.C.* Washington: National Gallery of Art, 1992.

Burford, A. *The Greek Temple Builders at Epidauros: A Social and Economic Study of Building in the Asklepian Sanctuary, during the Fourth and Early Third Centuries B.C..* Toronto: University of Toronto Press, 1969.

Burn, A.R. *The Lyric Age of Greece.* London: E. Arnold, 1960.

Burn, L. *Beazley Addenda: Additional References to A B V, A R V2 and Paralipomena.* Oxford: Oxford University Press for the British Academy, 1982.

Busignani, A. *Gli eroi di Riace: daimon e techne.* Florence: Sansoni, 1982.

Byl, S. *Recherches sur les grands traités biologiques d'Aristote: sources écrites et préjugés.* Brussels: Académie Royale de Belgique, 1980.

– "La vieillesse dans le Corpus hippocratique." *Colloque Lausanne* (1981): 85–95.

Carcopino, J. *La vie quotidienne à Rome à l'apogée de l'Empire.* Paris: Hachette, 1939.

Castiglioni, A. "Apothecary Jars in Antiquity." *Ciba Symposia* 6, no. 12 (1945): 2057.

Cherniss, H.F. *Aristotle's Criticism of Presocratic Philosophy.* New York: Octagon Books, 1964.

Chiaro, M. Del, ed. *Corinthiaca: Studies in Honor of Darrel A. Amyx.* Columbia: University of Missouri Press, 1986.

Childs, W.A.P. "The Classic as Realism in Greek Art." *Art Journal* 47, no. 1 (1988): 10–14.

Clark, K. *Another Part of the Wood: A Self-Portrait.* New York: Murray, 1974.

Clarke, E., and C.D. O'Malley. *The Human Brain and Spinal Cord: A Historical Survey Illustrated by Writings from Antiquity to the Twentieth Century.* Berkeley and Los Angeles: University of California Press, 1968.

La Collection hippocratique et son rôle dans l'histoire de la médecine: colloque de Strasbourg, 23–27 octobre 1972. Université des sciences humaines de Strasbourg. Travaux du Centre sur le Proche-Orient et la Grèce antiques, no. 2. Leyden: E.J. Brill, 1975.

Conacher, D.J. *Aeschylus' Prometheus Bound: A Literary Commentary.* Toronto: University of Toronto Press, 1980.

Cornford, F.M. *The Laws of Motion in Ancient Thought: An Inaugural Lecture.* Cambridge: Cambridge University Press, 1931.

Coulter, C.G., ed. *Greek Art, Archaic to Classical: A Symposium Held at the University of Cincinnati, April 2–3, 1982.* Cincinnati Classical Studies, new series, vol. 5. Leyden: E.J. Brill, 1985.

Daremberg, C. *La Médecine dans Homère.* Paris: Baillière, 1865.

Day, J.W. "Rituals in Stone: Early Greek Grave Epigrams and Monuments." *Journal of Hellenic Studies* 109 (1989): 16–28.

Dechend, H. von. "Il concetto di simmetria nelle culture arcaiche." In *La Simmetria,* edited by E. Agnazzi, 361–99. Bologna: Il Mulino, 1973.

Deichgräber, K. *Hippokrates De humoribus in der Geschichte der griechische Medizin.* Mainz-am-Rhein: Verlag der Akademie der Wissenschaften und der Literatur, 1972.

Demont, P. "Notes sur le récit de la pestilence athénienne chez Thucydide et sur ses rapports avec la médecine grecque de l'époque classique." *Colloque Lausanne* (1981): 341–54.

Diels, H., and W. Krantz, eds. *Fragmente der Vorsokratiker.* 7th ed. Berlin: Weidmann, 1951–54.

Diepolder, H. *Die attischer Grabreliefs des 5. und 4. Jahrhunderts v. Chr.* Darmstadt, 1965.

Diller, H. "Das Selbtverständnis der griechischen Medizin in der Zeit des Hippocrates." *Colloque Strasbourg* (1972): 77–93.

Dodds, E.R. *The Greeks and the Irrational.* Berkeley and Los Angeles: University of California Press, 1963.

Döring, K., and W. Kullmann, eds. *Studia Platonica: Festschrift für Hermann Gundert zu seinem 65. Geburtstag.* Amsterdam: Grüner, 1974.

Dover, K.J. *Greek Popular Morality in the Time of Plato and Aristotle.* Oxford: B. Blackwell, 1974.

Ducatillon, J. *Polémiques dans la Collection hippocratique.* Lille: Université de Lille III, Atelier Reproduction des thèses; Paris: Diffusion H. Champion, 1977.

– "Le traité des vents et la question hippocratique." *Colloque Lausanne* (1981): 263–76.

Duminil, M.P. "La description des vaisseaux dans les chapitres 11–19 du traité de la *Nature des os.*" *Colloque Paris* (1978): 135–47.

– *Le sang, les vaisseaux, le coeur dans la Collection hippocratique: anatomie et physiologie.* Paris: Les Belles Lettres, 1983.

Edelstein, L. *Ancient Medicine: Selected Papers of Ludwig Edelstein.* Edited by O. Temkin and C. Lillian Temkin. Translated by C. Lillian Temkin. Baltimore: Johns Hopkins Press, 1969.

– "The Dietetics of Antiquity." In *Ancient Medicine,* edited by O. Temkin and C. Lillian Temkin, translated by C. Lillian Temkin, 303–17. Baltimore: Johns Hopkins Press, 1969.

– "The Distinctive Hellenism of Greek Medicine." In *Ancient Medicine,* edited by O. Temkin and C. Lillian Temkin, translated by C. Lillian Temkin, 367–97. Baltimore: Johns Hopkins Press, 1969.

– *Die Geschichte der Sektion in der Antike: Quellen und Studien zur Geschichte der Naturwissenschaften und der Medizin* 3, no. 106. Berlin, 1922.

– *The Hippocratic Oath.* Baltimore: Johns Hopkins Press, 1943.

– "The Hippocratic Physician." In *Ancient Medicine*, edited by O. Temkin and C. Lillian Temkin, translated by C. Lillian Temkin, 87–110. Baltimore: Johns Hopkins Press, 1969.

– "The Professional Ethics of the Greek Physician." In *Ancient Medicine*, edited by O. Temkin and C. Lillian Temkin, translated by C. Lillian Temkin, 319–48. Baltimore: Johns Hopkins Press, 1969.

– "The Relation of Ancient Philosophy to Medicine." In *Ancient Medicine*, edited by O. Temkin and C. Lillian Temkin, translated by C. Lillian Temkin, 349–66. Baltimore: Johns Hopkins Press, 1969.

– Review and "Recent Trends in the Interpretation of Ancient Science." In *Ancient Medicine*, edited by O. Temkin and C. Lillian Temkin, translated by C. Lillian Temkin. 121–31, 401–39. Baltimore: Johns Hopkins Press, 1969.

Ehrenberg, V. *The People of Aristophanes: A Sociology of Old Attic Comedy.* Rev. ed. New York: Schocken Books, 1962.

Evans, E.C. *Physiognomics in the Ancient World.* Transactions of the American Philosophical Society, vol. 59, pt. 5. Philadelphia: American Philosophical Society, 1969.

Festugière, A.J. *Hippocrate: L'Ancienne Médecine.* Paris: Librairie C. Klincksieck, 1948.

Finley, M.I. "The Ancient City: from Fustel de Coulanges to Max Weber and Beyond." *Comparative Studies in Society and History* 19 (1977): 305–27.

– *The Olympic Games: The First Thousand Years.* London: Chatto and Windus, 1976.

Flashar, H. *Melancholie und Melancholiker in den medizinishchen Theorien der Antike.* Berlin: W. de Gruyter, 1966.

– ed. *Antike Medizin.* Darmstadt: Darmstadt Wissenschaftliche Buchges, 1971.

Formes de pensée dans la Collection hippocratique: Actes du IVe Colloque internationale hippocratique, Lausanne, 21–26 septembre 1981. Université de Lausanne, Publications de la Faculté des lettres, no. 26. Edited by F. Lasserre and P. Mudry. Geneva: Librairie Droz, 1983.

Formigli, E. "La tecnica di costruzione delle statue di Riace." In *Due bronzi da Riace: rinvenimento, restauro, analisi ed ipotesi d'interpretazione*, vol. 1, edited by L.V. Borelli and P. Pelagatti, 107–45. Rome: Istituto poligrafico e zecca dello Stato, 1984.

Fowler, B.H. "The Centaur's Smile: Pindar and the Archaic Aesthetic." In *Ancient Greek Art and Iconography*, edited by W.G. Moon, 159–70. Madison: University of Wisconsin Press, 1983.

Fuchs, W. "Zu den Grossbronzen von Riace." *Boreas* 4 (1981): 25–8.

Furley, D.J. "Self-Movers." In *Aristotle on Mind and the Senses: Proceedings of the the Seventh Symposium Aristotelicum, 1975*, edited by G.E.R. Lloyd and G.E.L. Owen, 165–79. Cambridge: Cambridge University Press, 1978.

– and J.S. Wilkie. *Galen on Respiration and the Arteries*. Princeton: Princeton University Press, 1984.

Fustel de Coulanges, N. *La cité antique*. Paris: Hachette, [1869]; reprint, Paris: Hachette, 1963.

Garland, R. *The Greek Way of Death*. Ithaca: Cornell University Press, 1985.

Gershenson, D.E., and D.A. Greenberg. *Anaxagoras and the Birth of Physics*. New York: Blaisdell Publishing Company, 1964.

Gill, B. *Here at the New Yorker*. New York: Random House, 1975.

Goldsmith, O. *The Vicar of Wakefield*. Dublin: W. & W. Smith, 1766.

Griefenhagen, A. *Corpus vasorum antiquorum: Deutschland*. Vol. 2. Berlin: Akademie-Verlag, 1983.

Guralnick, E. "Profiles of Kouroi." *American Journal of Archaeology* 89, no. 3 (1985): 399–409.

– "Proportions of *Kouroi*." *American Journal of Archaeology* 82 (1978): 461–72.

Guthrie, W.K.C. *A History of Greek Philosophy*. 3 vols. Cambridge: Cambridge University Press, 1962– .

Hall, T.S. *Ideas of Life and Matter: Studies in the History of General Physiology: 600 B.C.–1900 A.D.*. Vol. 1. Chicago: University of Chicago Press, 1969.

Hallett, C.H. "The Origins of the Classical Style in Sculpture." *Journal of Hellenic Studies* 106 (1986): 71–84.

Halperin, D.M., J.J. Winkler, and F.I. Zeitlin, eds. *Before Sexuality: The Construction of Erotic Experience in the Ancient Greek World*. Princeton: Princeton University Press, 1990.

Hands, A.R. *Charities and Social Aid in Greece and Rome*. London: Thames and Hudson, 1968.

Hanson, E.A. "The Medical Writers' Woman." In *Before Sexuality: The Construction of Erotic Experience in the Ancient Greek World*, edited by D.M. Halperin, J.J. Winkler, and F.I. Zeitlin, 309–37. Princeton: Princeton University Press, 1990.

Hardie, W.F.R. "Aristotle's Treatment of the Relation between Body and Soul." *Philosophical Quarterly* 14 (1964): 53–72.

Harris, C.R.S. *The Heart and the Vascular System in Ancient Greek Medicine: From Alcmaeon to Galen*. Oxford: Clarendon Press, 1973.

Harris, W.V. *Ancient Literacy*. Cambridge: Harvard University Press, 1989.

Harrison, E.B. "Early Classical Sculpture: the Bold Style." In *Greek Art, Archaic to Classical: A Symposium Held at the University of Cincinnati, April 2–3, 1982*, edited by C.G. Coulter, 40–65. Leyden: E.J. Brill, 1985.

Harvey, F.D. "Literacy in the Athenian Democracy." *Revue des études grecques* 29 (1966): 585–635.

Heinimann, F. *Nomos und Physis*. Basel: F. Reinhardt, 1945; reprint, Darmstadt, 1972.

Heintze, H. von. "Ein unbekanntes Augustusbildnis." In *In Memoriam Otto J. Brendel: Essays in Archaeology and the Humanities*, edited by L. Bonfante and H. von Heintze, 143–54. Mainz-am-Rhein: P. von Zabern, 1976.

Helbig, W. *Führer durch die öffentlichen Sammlungen Klassischer Altertümer in Rom*. 4th ed. Edited by H. Speier. 4 vols. Tübingen: E. Wasmuth, 1963– .

Henschen, F. *The History of Diseases*. Translated by J. Tate. London: Longmans, 1966.

Hippocratica: Actes du Colloque hippocratique de Paris, 4–9 septembre 1978. Colloques internationaux du Centre national de la recherche scientifique, no. 583. Edited by M.D. Grmek. Paris: Éditions du Centre national de la recherche scientifique, 1980.

Hölscher, T. *Ideal und Wirklichkeit in den Bildnissen Alexanders des Grossen*. Heidelberg: C. Winter, 1971.

Hollander, A. *Seeing through Clothes*. New York: Viking Press, 1978.

Houser, C. "The Riace Marina Bronze Statues, Classical or Classicizing?" *Source* 1 (1982): 1–11.

Humphreys, S.C. *Anthropology and the Greeks*. London: Routledge and Kegan Paul, 1978.

Hunter, V. "Classics and Anthropology." *Phoenix* 35, no. 2 (1981): 25–31.

Hurwit, Jeffrey M. *The Art and Culture of Early Greece, 1100–480 B.C.* Ithaca: Cornell University Press, 1985.

– "The Kritios Boy: Discovery, Reconstruction and Date." *American Journal of Archaeology* 93, no. 1 (1989): 41–80.

Immerwahr, H.R. *Attic Scripts: A Survey*. Oxford: Clarendon Press, 1990.

Ioannidi, H. "Les notions de partie du corps et d'organe." *Colloque Lausanne* (1981): 327–30.

Irigoin, J. "La formation du vocabulaire de l'anatomie en grec: du mycénien aux principaux traités de la Collection hippocratique." *Colloque Strasbourg* (1972): 247–58.

Jaeger, W.W. *Paideia: the Ideals of Greek Culture*. 2d ed. Translated by G. Highet. 3 vols. New York: Oxford University Press, 1939–46.

– "Das Pneuma im Lykeion." *Hermes* 48 (1913): 31–70.

Johannowsky, W. "Una nuova replica della testa dell' 'Apollo dell'Omphalos' da Baia." *Annuario della Scuola archeologica di Atene e delle Missioni italiane in Oriente* 45–46, nos. 29–30 (1967–68): 373–9.

Jones, C.P. *Plutarch and Rome*. Oxford: Clarendon Press, 1971.

Jones, W.H.S. "Ancient Documents and Contemporary Life, with Special Reference to the Hippocratic *Corpus*, Celsus and Pliny." In *Science, Medicine and History: Essays on the Evolution of Scientific Thought and Medical Practice in Honour of Charles Singer*, vol. 1, edited by E. Ashworth Underwood, 101–10. London: Oxford University Press, 1953.

– *Malaria and Greek History: To Which Is Added the History of Greek Therapeutics and the Malaria Theory.* Manchester: Manchester University Press, 1909.

– *Philosophy and Medicine in Ancient Greece, with an Edition of "Periarchaies ietrikes."* Baltimore: Johns Hopkins Press, 1946.

– et al., eds. *Hippocrates.* 4 vols. Cambridge and London: Harvard University Press, 1923–88.

Jouanna, J. *Hippocrate: La Nature de l'homme.* Corpus Medicorum Graecorum, vol. 1, nos. 1, 3. Berlin: Akademie-Verlag, 1975.

– *Hippocrate: pour une archéologie de l'École de Cnide.* Paris: Les Belles Lettres, 1974.

Kahn, C.H. *The Art and Thought of Heraclitus: An Edition of the Fragments with Translation and Commentary.* Cambridge: Cambridge University Press, 1979.

– "Religion and Philosophy in Empedocles' Doctrine of the Soul." *Arciv für Geschichte der Philosophie* 42 (1960): 46–63.

Karakatsanis, P. *Studien zu archaischen Kolossalwerken.* Europäische Hochschulschriften 38, vol. 9. Frankfurt am Main: P. Lang, 1986.

Karouzos, C. *Aristodikos: Studien zur Geschichte der spätarchaisch-attischen Plastik und der Grabstatue.* Stuttgart: W. Kohlhammer, 1961.

Kenner, H. *Weinen und Lachen in der griechischen Kunst.* Vienna, 1960.

Kerferd, G.B. *The Sophistic Movement.* Cambridge: Cambridge University Press, 1981.

Kirk, G.S., J.E. Raven, and M. Schofield. *The Presocratic Philosophers: A Critical History with a Selection of Texts.* 2d ed. Cambridge: Cambridge University Press, 1983.

Kleemann, I. *Frühe Bewegung: Undersuchungen zur archäischen Form bis zum Aufkommen der Ponderation in der griechischen Kunst.* Vol. 1. Mainz-am-Rhein: P. von Zabern, 1984.

Klibansky, R., E. Panofsky, and F. Saxl. *Saturn and Melancholy: Studies in the History of Natural Philosophy, Religion and Art.* London: Nelson, 1964.

Koelbing, H.M. *Arzt und Patient in der antiken Welt.* Zurich: Artemis Verlag, 1977.

– "Le médecin hippocratique au lit du malade." *Colloque Paris* (1978): 321–32.

Kostoglou-Despoine, A. *Problemata tes Parianes Plastikes tou 5ou Aiona p. Ch.* Thessaloniki, 1979.

Kühn, D.C.G. *Claudii Galeni opera omnia.* Leipzig, 1821–26.

Kyle, D.G. *Athletics in Ancient Athens.* Leyden: E.J. Brill, 1987.

Lacey, W.K. *The Family in Classical Greece.* London: Thames and Hudson, 1968.

Lanata, G. *Medicina magica e religione popolare in Grecia fino all'età di Ippocrate.* Rome: Edizioni dell'Ateneo, 1967.

Langholf, V. *Medical Theories in Hippocrates: Early Texts and the "Epidemics."* Untersuchungen zur antiken Literatur und Geschichte. Berlin: W. de Gruyter, 1990.

– *Syntaktische Untersuchungen zu Hippokrates-Texten: Brachylogische Syntagmen in den individuellen Krankheits- Falbeschreibungen der hippokratischen Schriften-sammlung.* Mainz-am-Rhein: Akademie der Wissenschaften und der Literatur, 1977.

Leftwich, G. "Ancient Conceptions of the Body and the Canon of Polykleitos." Ph.D. diss., Princeton University, 1987.

Lexicon Iconographicum Mythologiae Classicae. Vol. 2. Zurich: Artemis, 1984.

Lichtenthaeler, C. *Le traité des vents est typiquement pseudo-hippocratique: Amicus Aristoteles, sed magis amica veritas: XIV étude hippocratique.* Études d'histoire de la médecine, 8. Geneva: Librairie Droz, 1991.

Littré, E. *Oeuvres complètes d'Hippocrate.* 10 vols. Paris: J.B. Baillière, 1849–61.

Lloyd, G.E.R. "The Definition, Status, and Methods of the Medical $T\acute{\epsilon}\chi\nu\eta$ in the Fifth and Fourth Centuries." *Science and Philosophy in Classical Greece*, edited by A.C. Bowen, 249–60. New York and London, 1991.

– *Demystifying Mentalities.* Cambridge: Cambridge University Press, 1990.

– *Magic, Reason and Experience: Studies in the Origins and Development of Greek Science.* Cambridge: Cambridge University Press, 1979.

– *Methods and Problems in Greek Science.* Cambridge: Cambridge University Press, 1991.

– *Polarity and Analogy: Two Types of Argumentation in Early Greek Thought.* Cambridge: Cambridge University Press, 1966.

– *The Revolutions of Wisdom: Studies in the Claims and Practice of Ancient Greek Science.* Berkeley and Los Angeles: University of California Press, 1988.

– *Science, Folklore and Ideology: Studies in the Life Sciences in Ancient Greece.* Cambridge: Cambridge University Press, 1983.

– and G.E.L. Owen, eds. *Aristotle on Mind and the Senses: Proceedings of the Seventh Symposium Aristotelicum, 1975.* Cambridge: Cambridge University Press, 1978.

Lombardi Satriani, L.M., and M. Paoletti, eds. *Gli eroi venuti dal mare [Heroes from the Sea].* Rome: Gangemi, 1986.

Longrigg, J. "(Hippocrates') *Ancient Medicine* and Its Intellectual Context." *Colloque Lausanne* (1981): 249–56.

– "Philosophy and Medicine: Some Early Interactions." *Harvard Studies in Classical Philology* 67 (1963): 147–75.

Lonie, I.M. *The Hippocratic Treatises "On Generation," "On the Nature of the Child," "Diseases IV": A Commentary.* Ars Medica: Texte und Untersuchungen zur Queleekunde der Alten Medizin, vol. 2, no. 7. Berlin: W. de Gruyter, 1981.

– "Literacy and the Development of Hippocratic Medicine." *Colloque Lausanne* (1981): 145–61.

Lorenz, T. *Polyklet.* Wiesbaden: F. Steiner, 1972.

Lullies, R., and M. Hirmer. *Greek Sculpture.* Rev. ed. New York: Harry N. Abrams, 1960.

MacCormack, S. *Art and Ceremony in Late Antiquity.* Berkeley and Los Angeles: University of California Press, 1981.

MacKinney, L. "The Concept of Isonomia in Greek Medicine." In *Isonomia:*

Studien zur Gleichheitsvorstellung im greichischen Denken, edited by J. Mau and E.G. Schmidt, 81–4. Berlin: Akademie Verlag, 1964.

McManus, I.C. "Scrotal Asymmetry in Man and in Ancient Sculpture." *Nature* 259, no. 5542 (1976): 21.

Maddalena, A. "L'aria di Anasimene come sintesi." *Atti del Reale Istituto veneto* 97, no. 2 (1938–39): 515–45.

– "Eraclito nell'interpretazione di Platone e d'Aristotole." *Atti del Reale Instituto di scienze, lettere ed arti* 98 (1939): 219–43.

Majno, G. *The Healing Hand.* Cambridge: Harvard University Press, 1975.

Maloney, G., P. Potter, and W. Frohn-Villeneauve, eds. *Concordance des oeuvres hippocratiques.* 5 vols. Montréal: Éditions du Sphinx, 1984.

Mansfeld, J. "Theoretical and Empirical Attitudes in Early Greek Scientific Medicine." *Colloque Paris* (1978): 371–92.

Marelli, C. "Place de la *Collection hippocratique* dans les théories biologiques sur le sommeil." *Colloque Lausanne* (1981): 331–40.

Martin, R. "Aspects financiers et sociaux des programmes de construction dans les villes grecques de Grande Grèce et de Sicile." In *Atti del XIIo Convegno sulla Magna Grecia. Taranto, 8–14 ottobre 1972,* 185–206. Naples: Arte tipografica, 1973.

Mattusch, C.C. *Greek Bronze Statuary: from the Beginnings through the Fifth Century* B.C. Ithaca: Cornell University Press, 1988.

Mau, J., and E.G. Schmidt, eds. *Isonomia: Studien zur Gleichheitsvorstellung im griechischen Denken.* Berlin: Akademie-Verlag, 1964.

Michel, D. *Alexander als Vorbild für Pompeius, Caesar und Marcus Antonius.* Latomus 94. Brussels: Latomus Revue d'études latines, 1967.

Mieli, A. "L'epoca dei sofisti e la personalità di Socrate." *Archeion* 11 (1929): 178–89.

Momigliano, A. In S.C. Humphreys, *Anthropology and the Greeks,* 58. London: Routledge and Kegan Paul, 1978.

Moon, W.G., ed. *Ancient Greek Art and Iconography.* Madison: University of Wisconsin Press, 1983.

Morsink, J. *Aristotle on the Generation of Animals: A Philosophical Study.* Washington: University Press of America, 1982.

Muri, W. "Melancholie und schwarze Galle." In *Antike Medizin,* edited by H. Flashar, 165–90. Darmstadt: Darmstadt Wissenschaftliche Buchges, 1971.

Nodelman, S. "How to Read a Roman Portrait." *Art in America* 63, no. 1 (1975): 26–33.

Nussbaum, M.C. *Aristotle's De Motu Animalium: Text with Translation, Commentary, and Interpretive Essays.* Princeton: Princeton University Press, 1978.

O'Brien, Denis. *Empedocles' Cosmic Cycle: A Reconstruction from the Fragments and Secondary Sources.* London: Cambridge University Press, 1969.

– *Theories of Weight in the Ancient World: Four Essays on Democritus, Plato and*

Aristotle: a Study in the Development of Ideas. 4 vols. Paris: Les Belles Lettres; Leyden: E.J. Brill, 1981–86.

Ohly, D. *Die Aegineten: Die Marmorskulpturen des Tempels der Aphaia auf Aegina.* Vol. 1, *Die Ostgiebelsgruppe.* Munich: Beck, 1976.

Onians, J. *Art and Thought in the Hellenistic Age: The Greek World View, 350–50 B.C.* London: Thames and Hudson, 1979.

Onians, R.B. *The Origins of European Thought about the Body, the Mind, the Soul, the World, Time, and Fate.* 2d ed. Cambridge: Cambridge University Press, 1988.

Onofrio, A.M. d'. *"Korai* e *kouroi* funerari attici." In *Archeologia e storia antica,* 4:135–70. Naples: Instituto universitario orientale, 1982.

Osborne, R.G. "Death Revisited; Death Revised. The Death of the Artist in Archaic and Classical Greece." *Art History* 11, no. 1 (1988): 1–16.

Ostwald, M. *Nomos and the Beginning of the Athenian Democracy.* Oxford: Clarendon Press, 1969.

Overbeck, J. *Die antiken Schriftquellen zur Geschichte der bildenden Kunst bei den Griechen.* Leipzig: Engelmann, 1868; reprint. Hildesheim: G. Olms, 1971.

Owen, G.E.L. *Logic, Science and Dialectic: Collected Papers in Greek Philosophy.* Edited by M. Nussbaum. Ithaca: Cornell University Press, 1986.

Pandermalis, D. "Sul programma della decorazione scultorea." In *La Villa dei Papiri: Secondo Supplemento a Cronache Ercolanese 13/1983,* 19–50. Napoli: G. Macchiaroli, 1983.

Paribeni, E. "Lo stile e la datazione [The Style and Dating]." In *Gli eroi venuti dal mare* [*Heroes from the Sea*], edited by L.M. Lombardi Satriani and M. Paoletti, 65–76. Rome: Gangemi, 1986.

Phillips, E.D. *Greek Medicine.* London: Thames and Hudson, 1973.

Pigeaud, J. *La maladie de l'âme: étude sur la relation de l'âme et du corps dans la tradition médico-philosophique antique.* Paris: Les Belles Lettres, 1981.

Pitrè, G. *Biblioteca delle tradizioni popolari siciliane.* Vol. 19, *Medicina popolare siciliana.* Turin: Clausen, 1896.

– *Sicilian Folk Medicine.* Translated by P.H. Williams. Lawrence, Kans.: University of Kansas Press, 1971.

Pollitt, J.J. *The Ancient View of Greek Art: Criticism, History, and Terminology.* New Haven: Yale University Press, 1974.

– *Art and Experience in Classical Greece.* Cambridge: Cambridge University Press, 1972.

– *The Art of Greece 1400–31 B.C.: Sources and Documents in the History of Art.* Edited by H.W. Janson. Englewood Cliffs: Prentice-Hall, 1965.

Poulsen, V.H. *Les portraits romains.* Vol. 1, *République et dynastie julienne.* Copenhagen: Ny Carlsberg Glyptothek, 1962.

– *Der strenge Stil: Studien zur Geschichte der griechischen Plastik 480–450 v. Chr.* Acta Archaeologica, no. 8. Copenhagen: Levin & Munksgaard, 1937.

Preisshofen, F. "Sokrates im Gesprach mit Parrhasios und Kleiton." In *Studia*

Platonica: Festschrift für Hermann Gundert zu seinem 65. Geburtstag, edited by K. Döring and W. Kullmann, 21–40. Amsterdam: Grüner, 1974.

Preziozi, D. *Minoan Architectural Design: Formation and Signification.* Berlin: Mouton, 1983.

Raven, J.E. "Polyclitus and Pythagoreanism." *Classical Quarterly* 45 (1951): 147–52.

Regnéll, Hans. *Ancient Views on the Nature of Life: Three Studies in the Philosophies of the Atomists, Plato and Aristotle.* Lund: Gleerup, 1967.

Richter, G.M.A. *Kouroi: Archaic Greek Youths: A Study of the Development of the Kouros Type in Greek Sculpture.* 3d ed. London: Phaidon, 1970.

– *The Portraits of the Greeks.* Rev. ed. Ithaca: Cornell University Press, 1984.

– *The Sculpture and Sculptors of the Greeks.* 4th ed. New Haven: Yale University Press, 1970.

Ridgway, B.S. *Fifth Century Styles in Greek Sculpture.* Princeton: Princeton University Press, 1981.

– "The Riace Bronzes: A Minority Viewpoint." In *Due bronzi da Riace: rinvenimento, restauro, analisi ed ipotesi d'interpretazione,* vol. 1, edited by L.V. Borelli and P. Pelagatti, 313–26. Rome: Istituto poligrafico e zecca dello Stato, 1984.

– *Roman Copies of Greek Sculpture: The Problem of the Originals.* Ann Arbor: University of Michigan Press, 1984.

– *The Severe Style in Greek Sculpture.* Princeton: Princeton University Press, 1970.

– "The State of Research on Ancient Art." *Art Bulletin* 48, no. 1 (1986): 7–23.

Rivier, A. "Sur le rationalisme des premiers philosophes grecs." *Revue de théologie et de philosophie* 5 (1955): 1–15.

Robertson, M. *A History of Greek Art.* 2 vols. London: Cambridge University Press, 1975.

Robinson, C.E. *Everyday Life in Ancient Greece.* Oxford: Clarendon Press, 1958.

Roselli, A. "Problemi relativi ai trattati chirurgici *De Fracturis* e *De Articulis.*" *Colloque Strasbourg* (1972): 229–33.

Roussel, M. "La notion de traction dans le *Corpus* hippocratique: vers une étude globale." *Colloque Lausanne* (1981): 423–6.

Russell, D.A. *Plutarch.* London: Duckworth, 1973.

Sabbione, C. "La statua A," "La statua B," and appendix. In *Due bronzi da Riace: rinvenimento, restauro, analisi ed ipotesi d'interpretazione,* vol. 1, edited by L.V. Borelli and P. Pelagatti, 157–225. Rome: Istituto poligrafico e zecca dello Stato, 1984.

Saunders, J.B. de C.M. *The Transitions from Ancient Egyptian to Greek Medicine.* Logan Clendening Lectures on the History and Philosophy of Medicine, 10th series. Lawrence, Kans.: University of Kansas Press, 1963.

Scarborough, J. *Facets of Hellenic Life.* Boston: Houghton Mifflin, 1976.

Schöner, E. *Das Vierschema in der antiken Humoralpathologie.* Sudhoffs Archiv für Geschichte der Medizin under der Naturwissenshaften, no. 4. Wiesbaden, 1964.

Schofield, M. *An Essay on Anaxagoras.* Cambridge: Cambridge University Press, 1980.

Schumacher, J. *Antike Medizin: Die naturphilosophischen Grundlagen der Medizin in der griechischen Antike.* 2d rev. ed. Berlin: W. de Gruyter, 1963.

Schweitzer, B. *Die Bildniskunst der römischen Republik.* Leipzig: Koehler & Amelang, 1948.

Schwingenstein, C. *Die Figurenaustattung des griechischen Theatergebäudes.* Münchner Archäologische Studien, vol. 8. Munich: Fink, 1977.

Sellers, E. *The Elder Pliny's Chapters on the History of Art.* Translated by K. Jex-Blake. London, 1896; reprint, Chicago: Argonaut, 1968.

Sena, C. "Fotogrammetria dei bronzi di Riace." In *Due bronzi da Riace: rinvenimento, restauro, analisi ed ipotesi d'interpretazione,* vol. 1, edited by L.V. Borelli and P. Pelagatti, 227–9. Rome: Istituto poligrafico e zecca dello Stato, 1984.

Serwint, N. "Greek Athletic Sculpture of the Fifth and Fourth Centuries B.C.: An Iconographic Study." Ph.D. diss., Princeton University, 1987.

Sigerist, H.E. *Civilization and Disease.* Ithaca: Cornell University Press, 1943.

– *A History of Medicine.* 2 vols. New York: Oxford University Press, 1951–61.

Smith, W.D. "The Development of Classical Dietetic Theory." *Colloque Paris* (1978): 439–48.

– *The Hippocratic Tradition.* Ithaca: Cornell University Press, 1979.

Snell, B. *The Discovery of the Mind.* Translated by T.G. Rosenmeyer. Oxford: Blackwell, 1953.

Solmsen, F. "Greek Philosophy and the Discovery of the Nerves." *Museum Helveticum* 19 (1961): 150–67.

– "Griechische Philosophie und die Entdeckung der Nerven." In *Antike Medizin,* edited by H. Flashar, 202–78. Darmstadt: Darmstadt Wissenschaftliche Buchges, 1971.

– "The Vital Heat, the Inborn *Pneuma,* and the Aether." *Journal of Hellenic Studies* 77 (1957): 119–23.

Sorabji, R.R.K. "Body and Soul in Aristotle." *Philosophy* 49 (1974): 63–89.

Sow, M. "Lecture du paragraphe I du traité hippocratique de la *Maladie sacrée* (ou *Epilepsie*) à la lumière de la médecine traditionelle africaine." *Colloque Lausanne* (1981): 121–8.

Sprague, R.K., ed. *The Older Sophists: A Complete Translation by Several Hands of the Fragments in "Die Fragmente der Vorsokratiker."* Columbia: University of South Carolina Press, 1972.

Steuben, H. von. *Der Kanon des Polyklet: Doryphoros und Amazone.* Tübingen: E. Wasmuth, 1973.

Stewart, A.F. "The Canon of Polykleitos: A Question of Evidence." *Journal of Hellenic Studies* 98 (1978): 122–31.

– *Greek Sculpture: An Exploration.* 2 vols. New Haven: Yale University Press, 1990.

– "Scrotal Asymmetry: An Appendix." *Nature* 262 (1976): 155.

– *Skopas of Paros.* Park Ridge, NJ: Noyes Press, 1977.

– "When Is a Kouros Not an Apollo? The Tenea 'Apollo' Revisited." In *Corinthiaca: Studies in Honor of Darrel A. Amyx*, edited by M. Del Chiaro, 54–70. Columbia: University of Missouri Press, 1986.

Strauss, Leo. *The City and Man*. Chicago: Rand McNally, 1964.

Svenbro, J. "A Mégara Hyblaea: le corps géomètre." *Annales: économies, sociétés, cultures* 37, nos. 5–6 (1982): 953–64.

Theiler, W. *Zur Geschichte der teleologischen Naturbetrachtung bis auf Aristoteles*. 2d ed. Berlin: W. de Gruyter, 1965.

Thivel, A. *Cnide et Cos?: essai sur les doctrines médicales dans la collection hippocratique*. Paris: Les Belles Lettres, 1981.

Thomas, R. *Athletenstatuetten des spätarchaik und des strengen Stils*. Archaeologica 18. Rome: G. Bretschneider, 1981.

Tobin, R. "The Canon of Polykleitos." *American Journal of Archaeology* 79 (1975): 307–21.

Tölle-Kastenbein, R. *Frühklassische Peplosfiguren: Originale*. Mainz-am-Rhein: P. von Zabern, 1980.

Totok, W. *Handbuch der Geschichte der Philosophie*. Vol. 1, *Altertum: Indische, Chinesische, Griechische-römische Philosophie*. Frankfurt am Main: V. Klostermann, 1964.

Underwood, E.A., ed. *Science, Medicine, and History: Essays on the Evolution of Scientific Thought and Medical Practice in Honour of Charles Singer*. Vol. 1. London: Oxford University Press, 1953.

Vatin, C. "Couroi argiens à Delphes." *Études delphiques: bulletin de correspondance héllenique* 4 (1977): 13–22.

– "Monuments votifs de Delphes." *Bulletin de correspondance héllenique* 106 (1982): 509–25.

Vegetti, M. "Metafora politica e immagine del corpo negli scritti ippocratici." *Colloque Lausanne* (1981): 459–70.

Verbeke, G. "Doctrine du Pneuma et entéléchisme chez Aristote." In *Aristotle on Mind and the Senses: Proceedings of the Seventh Symposium Aristotelicum, 1975*, edited by G.E.R. Lloyd and G.E.L. Owen, 191–213. Cambridge: Cambridge University Press, 1978.

Vermeule, E. *Aspects of Death in Early Greek Art and Poetry*. Berkeley and Los Angeles: University of California Press, 1979.

Vernant, J.-P. "Remarques sur les formes et les limites de la pensée technique chez les Grecs." *Revue d'histoire des sciences et de leurs applications* 10 (1957): 205–25.

Vierneisel, K., and P. Zanker, eds. *Die Bildnisse des Augustus: Herrcherbild und Politik in kaiserlichen Rom*. Munich: Beck, 1979.

Vierneisel-Schlörb, B. *Klassische Skulpturen des 5. und 4. Jahrhunderts v. Chr.* Glypothek München, Katalog der Skulpturen. 2 vols. Munich: Beck, 1979.

Vikan, G. "Art, Medicine and Magic in Early Byzantium." *Dumbarton Oaks Papers* 38 (1984): 65ff.

Vita, A. di. "Due capolavori attici: gli oplitodromi-'eroi' di Riace." In *Due bronzi da Riace: rinvenimento, restauro, analisi ed ipotesi d'interpretazione*, vol. 2, edited by L.V. Borelli and P. Pelagatti, 251–76. Rome: Istituto poligrafico e zecca dello Stato, 1984.

Vlastos, G. "Isonomia." *American Journal of Philology* 74 (1953): 337–66.

Vostchinina, A. *Le portrait romain: album et catalogue illustré de toute la collection, Musée de l'Ermitage.* Leningrad: Éditions d'art Aurore, 1974.

Webster, T.B.L. *Art and Literature in Fourth Century Athens.* London: University of London, Athlone Press, 1956.

Weerts, E. *Plato und der Heraklitismus: ein Beitrage zum Problem der Historie im Platonischen Dialog.* Leipzig: Dieterich, 1931.

Wheelwright, P. *Heraclitus.* Princeton: Princeton University Press, 1959.

Wiersma, W. "Die aristotelische Lehre vom Pneuma." *Mnemosyne* 11 (1943): 102–7.

Wiesner, J. "The Unity of the *De Somno* and the Physiological Explanation of Sleep in Aristotle." In *Aristotle on Mind and the Senses: Proceedings of the Seventh Symposium Aristotelicum, 1975*, edited by G.E.R. Lloyd and G.E.L. Owen, 241–79. Cambridge: Cambridge University Press, 1978.

Wilson, A. *Anglo-Saxon Attitudes.* London: Secker & Warburg, 1959.

Wilson, E. *To the Finland Station: A Study in the Writing and Acting of History.* London: Secker & Warburg, 1940.

Winckelmann, J.J. *History of Ancient Art.* Translated by G.H. Lodge. 4 books in 2 vols. New York: F. Unger Publishing Co., 1968.

Winkes, R. "Physiognomonia: Probleme der Charakterinterpretation römischer Porträts." *Aufsteig und Niedergand* 1, no. 4 (1973): 899–926.

Woysch-Méautis, D. *La représentation des animaux et des êtres fabuleux sur les monuments funéraires grecs: de l'époque archaïque à la fin du IVe siècle.* Cahiers d'archéologie romande, no. 21. Lausanne: Bibliothèque historique vaudoise, 1982.

Wright, M.R., ed. *Empedocles: The Extant Fragments.* New Haven: Yale University Press, 1981.

Yalouris, N. "Die Anfänge der griechischen Porträtkunst und der Physiognomon Zopyros." *Antike Kunst* 29 (1986): 5–7.

Young, D.C. *The Olympic Myth of Greek Amateur Athletics.* Chicago: Ares Publishers, 1984.

Zinzerling, V. "Zum Bedeutungsgehalt des archaïschen Kuros." *Eirene* 13 (1975): 19–34.

Index Locorum

Index

Achilles (figure): and melancholia, 63, 124n2; as possible identity for *Doryphoros*, 71

Achilles (representation of), 93–4, 124n2

Achilles and the tortoise: and motion, 73

Acropolis. *See* Athens

Aegina: and Democedes of Croton, xiii; sculptures from temple of Aphaea at, 33, 114n1, 115n4, pl. 11

Aeneas (figure), 98

Aeneid. See Virgil

Aeschylus (poet), 30

agalma(ta), 70, 71; kouroi as, 70–1, 121n5; and poetry, 70–1, 121n5

Agias (representation of). *See* Delphi

Ajax (figure): and melancholia, 62

Alcmaeon of Croton (philosopher): on the *Kanon*, 120n52

Alexander the Great (figure): and *anastole*, 3, 4, 103n3; and Pompey, 3, 4

anastole, 3–5, 104n3; and Alexander the Great, 3, 4; and Augustus, 3, 104n3; and courage, 4–5; and Nero, 3; in

Physiognomics, 3, 5; Plutarch on, 3, 4; and Pompey, 3, 4

Anavysos, "Kroisos" from (sculpture): generalized identity of, 70, 117n18

Anaxagoras of Clazomenae (philosopher), xii, xiii, 95, 96, 123n29; on anatomy, xiii, 80, 82, 83, 88; at Athens, 22, 30, 73, 74, 78, 79; on blood, 82; on *contrapposto*, 79–80, 82–3; on cosmology, 73–6 passim, 122n14; on facial expression, 89–90; on hands, 22, 54, 78, 79, 89; on human uniqueness, 54, 89–90; influence of, on Aristotle, 81, 82, 89–90; influence of, on sculpture, 79–80, 83; on motion, 66, 73–84 passim, 121n12; on *nous*, 30, 73; as "Nous," 73; and Pneumatic theory of the soul, 44, 48, 66, 69. *See also* Sophists

Anaximenes of Miletus (philosopher): on Pneumatic soul, 44

Anchises (figure), 98

animating forces, 17, 30–1,

58, 66, 68, 88, 91; and blood vessels, 49; and *contrapposto*, 83; and *dike*, 30; in Girl from Paros, 59; Hippocratic physicians on, 50, 60; and inhalation, 59; and motion, 69, 76, 82–4, 91, 92, 96; natural philosophy on, xiii, 59; in Omphalos Apollo, 58, 59, 68; pre-Socratic thought on, 31, 59; and respiration, 92; in Riace warriors, 58, 59; and the soul, 49, 113n32. *See also* soul

Aphaea, temple of, at Aegina. *See* Aegina

Apollo
- Choiseul-Gouffier (sculpture), 32
- Omphalos (sculpture), ix, 32, 33, 58, fig. 1, pls. 1–2; animating forces in, 58, 59, 68; and Apollo Choiseul-Gouffier, 32; and Aristodikos, 41; arms in, 32, 41, 42, 51, 53, 54–5; blood vessels in, 32, 33, 36, 37, 49, 51–60 passim, 115n4; *contrapposto* in, 32, 37, 39, 40, 41, 42, 80; as experimental statue, 68;